Harry the Hypno-potamus
More Metaphorical Tales for Children
Volume 2

Linda Thomson PhD MSN CPNP

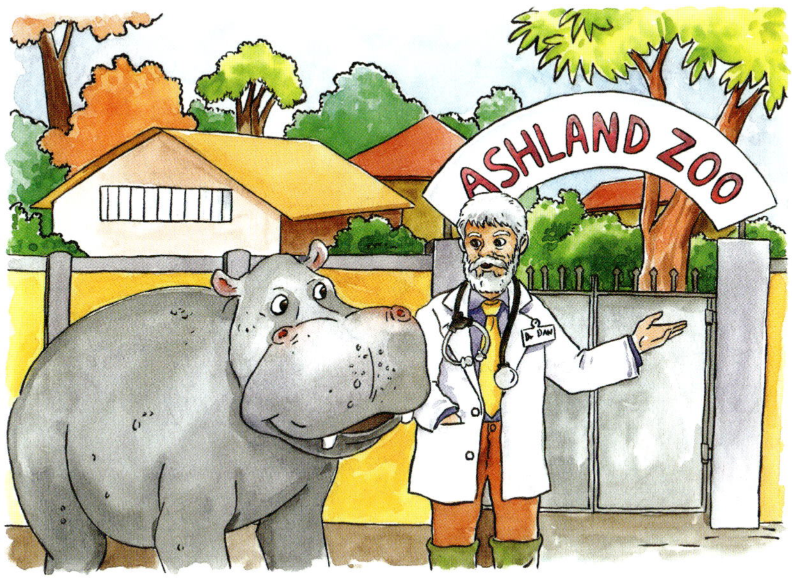

Crown House Publishing Limited
www.crownhouse.co.uk – www.crownhousepublishing.com

First published by

Crown House Publishing Ltd
Crown Buildings, Bancyfelin, Carmarthen, Wales, SA33 5ND, UK
www.crownhouse.co.uk

and

Crown House Publishing Company LLC
6 Trowbridge Drive, Suite 5, Bethel, CT 06801, USA
www.crownhousepublishing.com

British Library of Cataloguing-in-Publication Data
A catalogue entry for this book is available from the British Library.

International Standard Book Number 978-184590117-2

Library of Congress Control Number 2008922773

Printed and bound by
Replika Press Pvt. Ltd, India

To George who has shared his heart, his life, and his love with me for 35 years.
He taught me that even more amazing than the magic of imagination is the power of love.

Contents

Pain

Other uses of hypnosis

Acknowledgments

If I can touch the stars, it is because I stand on the shoulders of giants. Everyone who uses hypnosis learned it from someone else. Many people have taught me about how to use hypnosis, and guided me as I was learning.

Flowing from my heart and mind, infusing these metaphorical tales with their actual words, are the thoughts and ideas of many remarkable clinicians. I am grateful for these gifts and freely pass them on to others so that they, too, can help children to help themselves.

David Gottsegen, MD, introduced me to the practice of using hypnosis in primary care pediatrics. I am eternally grateful.

Haley LaPlatte (Haley) and Conor Thomson (Conor) are my precious grandchildren and are the inspiration of my imagination.

Daniel P. Kohen, MD, (Dr. Dan) is a behavioral pediatrician. He has generously shared with many people, including myself, the wisdom gained from his vast experience in using hypnosis with children. With his co-author, Karen Olness, MD, Dr. Kohen wrote *Hypnosis and Hypnotherapy with Children*. Dan is a dear friend and amazing mentor. Moreover, he has quite a distinguished beard.

Gabor Filo, DDS, (Gabor) is the "Canadian guy" and a dentist. He has quite a memorable handlebar moustache.

Moshe Torem, MD, (Moshe) is a psychiatrist and founder of a center for mind–body medicine.

Phil Accaria, PhD, (Accaria) is a psychologist and past president of the American Society of Clinical Hypnosis.

Peter Bloom, MD, (Bloom) is a psychiatrist and past president of the International Society of Hypnosis.

Elvira Lang, MD, (Elvira) is an interventional radiologist whose research on helping patients through invasive procedures is known and respected throughout the world.

Meg Zweiback, MSN, CPNP, (Meg) is a pediatric nurse practitioner who does amazing therapeutic work with young children and their families.

William Wester, EdD, (Wester) is a psychologist. With Lawrence Sugarman, MD, Dr. Wester is the co-author of *Therapeutic Hypnosis with Children and Adolescents*. He also co-edited, with Donald O'Grady, PhD, *Clinical Hypnosis with Children*.

Sam Migdole, EdD, (Sam) is a psychologist and past president of both the New England Society of Clinical Hypnosis and the American Board of Psychological Hypnosis.

"Lex" is an amazing youngster who overcame his fear of toileting and created the metaphor of Squirt, the Shy Pumper Fire Truck.

Jacki Irland, MD, (Irland) is an obstetrician who uses hypnosis to help her patients deliver their babies in safety and comfort.

David Alter, PhD, (Alter) is a psychologist and member of the Executive Committee of the American Society of Clinical Hypnosis.

Joseph Zastrow, MD, (Joe) is a family practice physician who incorporates hypnosis into his medical practice.

Steve Gurgevich, PhD, (Gurg) is a psychologist who specializes in mind–body and behavioral medicine.

Ashley Goodman, DDS, (Dr. Goodman) is a dentist and vice-president of the American Board of Hypnosis in Dentistry.

Carol Ginandes, PhD, (Carol) is a researcher and master teacher of mind–body healing. Carol Low, PsyD (Carol) is a psychologist who has served in leadership positions in local and national hypnosis societies.

Michael Yapko, PhD, (Yapko) is a psychologist who is partial to pachyderms after being asked by the San Diego Wild Animal Park to use his skills as a clinician to help the endangered African and Asian elephant-breeding program.

George Glaser, MSW (George) is a giant in the world of hypnosis—both literally and figuratively.

Jud Reaney, MD, (Jud) is a pediatrician who combines hypnosis with biofeedback to help children help themselves. He is on the hypnosis faculty for the Society of Developmental and Behavioral Pediatrics.

Richard Kluft, MD (Kluft) is a psychiatrist who is well-known for his work with patients with dissociative identity disorders.

Steve Kahn, PhD, (Kahn) is a psychologist and president of the Society for Clinical and Experimental Hypnosis.

Howard Hall, PhD, (Howard) is a pediatric psychologist and an amazing pianist. He is on the hypnosis faculty for the Society of Developmental and Behavioral Pediatrics.

Steven Paulker, MD, (Paulker) is a cardiologist and past president of the Society of Medical Decision Making.

Melanie Gold, DO, (Goldie) is an adolescent medicine specialist. She is on the hypnosis faculty for the Society of Developmental and Behavioral Pediatrics.

Leora Kuttner, PhD, (Leora) is a psychologist and film maker who produced *No Tears, No Fears*. She is on the hypnosis faculty for the Society of Developmental and Behavioral Pediatrics.

Many Marks have made their mark on the world of hypnosis. I am especially grateful to Mark Geer, EdD, psychologist; Mark Weisberg, PhD, psychologist; Mark Adams, MSW, clinical social worker; and Mark Tracten, publisher of Crown House Publishing Limited who has been an enormous support in bringing Harry Hypno-potamus to the world.

Amir Raz, MD, (Raz) is a brilliant scientist who is helping to shed light on how hypnosis affects the brain. He has the energy of ten men.

George Thomson, MA, (Mr. Thomson) is my beloved husband and an elementary school principal extraordinaire.

Eric Willmarth, PhD, (Eric) is a psychologist who integrates hypnosis and biofeedback. In front of the camera, Eric has appeared as Elvis. Behind the camera he has made an incredible contribution to the field of hypnosis by filming a video history of international hypnosis experts.

Rebecca Kajander, MPH, CPNP, (Becky) is a pediatric nurse practitioner who combines biofeedback and hypnosis in her work with children. With Timothy Culbert, MD, (Tim) Becky co-authored *Be the Boss of your Body*. Tim helped to develop the Freeze Framer stress management system.

Ran Anbar, MD, (Ran) is a pediatric pulmonologist, researcher and prolific writer.

Steve Lankton, MSW, (Lankton) is a clinical social worker and editor of the American Journal of Hypnosis.

Carolyn Daitch, PhD, is a psychologist and author of *Affect Regulation Tool Box: Practical and Effective Hypnotic Interventions for the Overreactive Client*.

Da-Shih Hu, MD, (Da-Shih) is a psychiatrist. Many patients with non-epileptic seizures have been helped with Dr. Hu's hypnosis.

Harvey Zarren, MD, (Harvey) is a cardiologist and medical director of Healing the Heart Program.

Don Moss, PhD, (Dr. Moss) is a psychologist and editor of *Biofeedback*.

John "Jack" Watkins, PhD, (Jack) is a nonagenarian and a psychologist. With his wife, Helen, Dr. Watkins developed the specific theory of ego-state therapy.

Adam Keating, MD, (Adam) is a young pediatrician who helps his patients help themselves with hypnosis.

Chuck Burbridge, PhD, (Burbie) is a psychologist and editor of the American Society of Clinical Hypnosis Newsletter.

Maggie Phillips, PhD, (Maggie) is a psychologist who uses energy therapies in mind–body healing. She is the author of *Finding the Energy to Heal*.

Akira Otani, EdD, (Akira) is a psychologist, gifted clinician and amazing teacher.

Angela MacKenzie, MD, (Kenzie) is a pediatrician and friend from Down Under.

Sally Freeman, (Sally) editor of both my Harry Tales books, has been a joy to work with. As we sent manuscripts back and forth over the Internet, preparing *Harry* for press, I learned a lot about editing and Sally learned a lot about hypnosis and hypnotic language. I am grateful for all her help and advice.

Foreword

by Daniel P. Kohen, MD

This is Linda Thomson's second book of enchanting and healing stories about that wise and wonderful Hypno-potamus, Harry, who helps children to help themselves. Since the Harry Tales first appeared in 2005, parents, children, and their doctors and therapists have eagerly anticipated this latest volume.

As we noted in the foreword to the first *Harry the Hypno-potamus*, Linda Thomson is an accomplished, committed, and creative pediatric nurse practitioner who shares her experience and thoughtful sensitivity with us. With this second book of stories and adventures about the animals of the Ashland Zoo, she has done it again. She shows us how each animal, in its own unique way, cultivates imagination toward self-healing and resolving problems.

As in the first Harry volume, this one begins with a guide for pediatricians and other child health and mental health professionals. After a brief description of hypnosis, the author goes on to describe and explain metaphors—the cornerstone of each story. She outlines the categories of problems she will address including anxiety, unwanted habits, pain, and a miscellaneous but important group of common childhood challenges that range from undergoing a medical check-up to adapting to foster care.

We clinicians have enjoyed using the stories from the first Harry Tales to help children to help themselves, and to help parents help their children. The Harry stories stimulated our own creativity, and inspired us to develop other stories. Meanwhile, we encouraged parents and children to develop their own stories to facilitate healing and resolve problems.

We have wondered about other common childhood problems, and hoped that Harry the Hypno-potamus and his pal, Dr. Dan, the zoo veterinarian, might come up with some new ideas. Indeed they have! We are relieved to see that in this second book, the author, with Harry and Dr. Dan's help, has provided stories for a wide variety of anxiety problems, from fears of trying something new (as experienced by Moshe the Hoatzin, a South American bird afraid to leave his nest and fly), to general anxiety (Accaria Octopus), to Wester Wallaby's fear of heights, Sam Orangutan's worries about learning to use the toilet, and Irland Stork's difficulty swallowing pills.

In addition, the author provides an expanded approach to habit problems that include Gurgevich Gibbon's finger sucking, Carol the Kinkajou's habit cough, and cyclical vomiting and fear of vomiting as experienced and resolved by Kluft Turkey Vulture, who had a habit of throwing up, and Kahn Quetzal, who had a fear of throwing up.

Children's increasingly common and current problems are highlighted with wonderfully creative therapeutic stories that address feelings of sadness (Burbridge Kookaburra, who has trouble figuring out how to be happy), depression (Harvey Hyena who is so sad), ADHD (Raz Ratel who gets a special pill for his jeep), and coping with bullies (which Akira Okapi learns to do by finding out how to fit in). Anger management, recurrent abdominal pain, headaches, selective mutism, and managing pain during hospitalization are all also presented through stories of how various animals from the zoo help themselves to cope.

As a bonus, readers young and old, clinician and parent alike, learn interesting and accurate information about a variety of animals—familiar and unfamiliar, common and exotic.

I was very relieved to see that, in the process of helping Gabor the Beluga Whale overcome fears such as masks and beards, my namesake, Dr. Dan, decided in this volume to grow a beard so that he could best express his own personal story.

Like the first Harry Tales, this book is a lot of fun. It allows children and their families to utilize their natural skills of creative imagination and self-hypnosis in order to participate in their own healing and wellness. My patients, their families, and I are grateful to the trio of Linda Thomson, Harry the Hypno-potamus, and veterinarian Dr. Dan for their ongoing contribution to children's health. I wonder when the third book of Harry Tales will appear?

Daniel P. Kohen, MD
September 2007

Preface

Imagination is a gift you give yourself in the present that allows you to go into the future feeling better and stronger, more calm and comfortable.

I wrote the first Harry Hypno-potamus book for pediatric health and mental health professionals who were trained in hypnotherapy and experienced in child development. However, I soon discovered that clinicians who work with adults were also utilizing the stories with patients/clients. Parents, school teachers, and other professionals not trained in hypnosis were using the metaphors with children. Meanwhile, the children themselves were picking up the book to read about a shy turtle, an anxious elephant, a meerkat who wet the bed, a chimp who sucked his thumb, and other entertaining and educational tales.

Therefore, the second book of Harry Tales is for readers of all ages who want to learn what they never knew they knew and control what they never knew they could. It is for anyone who wants to learn relaxation skills and self-regulatory strategies in order to cope with pain, anxiety, habit disorders, and other physical and emotional problems. The Harry Tales are for clinicians who want to put the "care" back in health care, and are passionate about helping patients/clients live happier, more comfortable lives.

Sometimes it is difficult to believe that I actually get paid to work hypnotically with children because it is such a joy. They bring to me far more than I could ever give to them. Their spontaneous creativity is a treasure. The most amazing and effective metaphors are the ones the children create themselves. The story of Sam, the orangutan, contains a metaphor about a shy pumper fire truck that was created by a remarkable four-year-old boy. Truly, the solution to his problem was within, and he was able to access that ability through metaphor. I am grateful to him for sharing the story of Squirt with me, and for allowing me to share it with you.

It has been a pleasure to write these tales for children and adults. What gives me the greatest joy is learning that one of my stories has made a difference in the life of a child. As you utilize these stories in your work, I would be grateful if you would share with me any special experiences that you have had in using the tales. If, in your work, a child has created an amazing metaphor and would like to share with others in a third volume of Harry Tales, please send it to me, with their permission, at Linda.Thomson@Hitchcock.org

Enjoy!

Clinical Section

Introduction

The second book of *Harry the Hypno-potamus* tales contains metaphors that deal with a variety of physical and behavioral problems. Embedded in many of the metaphors are hypnotherapeutic techniques that can be used as part of a comprehensive approach to diagnosing and treating certain disorders.

Reading a child the first story, "Harry Tells Haley and Conor about Hypnosis," is a wonderful way to introduce a child to hypnosis and the power of imagination. Two metaphors in the book— a tale about a loon, and another about a hippopotamus and a tortoise— are based on real animals and life events. The rest of the events and their metaphors take place in the imaginary Ashland Zoo. There Dr. Dan, a wise and wonderful veterinarian, cares for all the animals. The animal character in each story has a physical or emotional problem, and learns specific hypnotherapeutic techniques and self-regulatory strategies to help master it. Most of the stories contain interesting zoological facts about the animal in the metaphor.

A story may be shared with a child who has that particular problem, or the techniques embedded in the metaphor can be applied to other situations, and adapted to other patients and clients. The developmental age of the child must always be considered. Some of the stories may fascinate a young child, yet contain techniques that are more appropriate for an older one. Some of the stories contain hypnotic scripts. In hypnosis, pacing, leading, cadence, rhythm, and vocal inflections are all important.

Pediatric Hypnosis

Imagining and pretending are integral to children's play. Hypnosis is a natural extension of employing fantasy to change or avoid an unpleasant situation, gratify unmet needs, remember the past, or invent the future. Hypnotherapeutic work enhances and strengthens the child's natural inclinations toward fantasy and creativity, exploration, and forming social relationships. Children strive to achieve self-efficacy and self-mastery, and they are generally receptive to hypnotic tools that will help them experience success.

The therapeutic alliance, or rapport, between child and clinician is critically important to the success of a hypnotic intervention. The child must feel safe, comfortable, and confident that he can trust the professional. Other important variables include the child's motivation to change, his expectation of success, and his active participation in the process.

Metaphorical Approaches

Throughout the ages, in all cultures around the world, parents have used stories to teach their children important life lessons. Children love stories and using their imagination. Our memories of childhood are filled with parables about compassion, courage and wisdom, stories of honesty and industriousness, and tales of mythical heroes and heroines. "The Little Engine That Could" and "The Hare and the Tortoise" taught us about perseverance. "The Ugly Duckling" taught us how deceptive appearances can be.

By using symbolic language and characters, metaphors convey their meaning indirectly. They open up a world of possibilities and experiences, stimulate curiosity, and expand horizons.

Symbolic language implies something more than its obvious or immediate meaning. The right brain processes symbolic language, subjective and sensory sensations; hypnosis is a right brain phenomenon that cultivates imagination. Metaphor may well be the language of the right brain, and it can be used very effectively in hypnotherapy.

A hypnotherapist uses metaphors to communicate simultaneously with both the conscious and the unconscious minds. The conscious mind processes the words, the narrative, and the ideas, while the therapeutic message is slipped into the unconscious via implication and connotation. The unconscious mind explores the broader meaning and the personalized relevance that gives the metaphor its potency. When a clinician skilled in hypnotherapy uses metaphors, the moral of the story is never explained, as they are in Aesop's fables. The impact of the tale is much more powerful when the individual figures out the personal relevance and meaning for herself.

The goal of the metaphor is to expand human consciousness through a right brain encounter linking emotion, symbolic language, and life experience.

In the 1960s, neurosurgeons Vogel and Bogen performed an unprecedented experimental surgical procedure on a patient with epilepsy: they intentionally severed the corpus collosum, the nerve pathways between the two hemispheres of the brain. As a result, scientists discovered that the right and left sides of the brain each has a unique way of handling information.

Although the two brain hemispheres receive information cooperatively, each has its individual style of dealing with what it receives. For example, the left brain works logically and literally on the sequential decoding of the printed word as the right brain simultaneously processes language in a holistic, implicative, and imagistic fashion. In other words, the left brain arranges all the puzzle pieces in order, while the right brain interprets the picture created by the separate pieces. While the left brain processes literal meaning, the right brain uses implication based on life experience to understand the whole picture. Generating imagery and gleaning the meaning of a story are right brain functions.

Metaphor appears to be the language of the right brain. This hemisphere is more involved in interpreting subjective and sensory experiences. Therefore, when communication is metaphorical, the right hemisphere is activated. Since psychosomatic symptoms are mainly generated by right brain functions, psychosomatic illness may be a right brain expression.

The metaphor allows a hypnotherapist to communicate symbolically with the unconscious mind. Because the right hemisphere mediates both symptomatology and metaphorical meaning, metaphorical approaches to therapy may be much less time-intensive. It is the right brain that comprehends metaphor; using metaphors in hypnosis may be a means of communicating directly with the right brain in its own language.

Using metaphors in hypnosis can bring about positive change. A therapeutic suggestion may not be obvious to the listener because it is so cleverly entwined and embedded in the story that she is unconsciously influenced to effect change without being consciously admonished to do so. As a result, the child may experience a sense of accomplishment and greater self-confidence. Metaphors may expose a child to new possibilities, new perspectives, and differing philosophies. Because they are subjectively experienced, metaphors help to bypass resistance. The child views the problem as something that is happening to somebody else; therefore, she does not feel personally threatened.

Inputting a positive message to the unconscious is only one function of the metaphor. They also replenish the soul. Because metaphors are non-threatening, they often engage and enhance empowerment, causing children to stretch their minds, broaden their horizons, and develop wisdom. By altering the individual's usual way of thinking, metaphors help to change his patterns of behavior.

Restating a child's problem in a non-threatening metaphor provides the patient with a different view of the situation. Reframing helps him to take charge of mastering or resolving the problem. In reframing, the facts of a situation or an event remain the same, but the way a child views or conceptualizes the situation changes, thereby altering the entire meaning. Sometimes it is necessary for the child to use other senses, or perceptions different from the ones he would ordinarily use to experience success. Metaphorical approaches encourage the child's unconscious mind to develop novel ways to overcome limitations.

Children love stories; they love to imagine and pretend. Hypnotherapeutic work enhances and strengthens a child's natural strivings toward exploration, social relationships, fantasy, and creativity. Cultivating a child's imagination through hypnotic metaphors is not only appealing, it is effective.

The metaphors in this book can ignite a child's creative imagination. Very young children may not need to figure out the meaning of the metaphor; rather, they immerse themselves in the fanciful tale and become intimately connected to the sensory experience. The child's simplistic and intuitive grasp of situations allows her to be open to the symbolic dimension and diversion of the experience. When a child is fully immersed in the story, her personal internal negative dialogue may be suppressed, and new possibilities can flourish. The child can make a personal connection with the character's situation or problem. By recognizing the personal relevance of the teaching tale, the child may discover a solution to her problem, thus enhancing her self-esteem and self-mastery.

The use of metaphors in hypnotherapy is certainly not limited to children. In their book *Therapeutic Metaphors for Children and the Child Within*, Mills and Crowley discuss metaphor's potential for creative reframing and unconscious learning in people of all ages. Most adults associate storytelling with pleasant childhood memories. According to Nick Owen in *The Magic of Metaphor*, "Stories connect the past with the present, and project both past and present into the future. Connecting between times and contexts, between ideas and concepts, between behaviors and values, stories enable the listeners to review and anticipate thought and action."

Listening to therapeutic tales effortlessly takes the individual into his inner world, stimulating unconscious restructuring, evoking his own solution to problems, and activating forces for change and healing. The metaphor's creative force can stimulate each person's unique inner processes, abilities, and resources. Using metaphor and helping the patient to create his own therapeutic tales can be an incredibly powerful tool in hypnosis.

Anxiety

The most commonly occurring mental disorder in children is anxiety. This disorder may have a specific cause, or it can be more generalized,

---

Mills, Joyce C., and Crowley, Richard J. *Therapeutic Metaphors for Children and The Child Within*. New York: Brunner/Mazel, 1986.
Owen, Nick. *The Magic of Metaphor*. Carmarthen, UK: Crown House Publishing, 2001

without an objective focus. Anxiety results from a real or perceived danger, or a threat to safety. Some anxiety is appropriate, necessary, and universal. It is a normal protective mechanism that heightens awareness and the ability to react to danger or a threatening situation. The difference between appropriate anxiety and anxiety as a mental disorder is a matter of degree.

Some children live in a state of hyper-arousal which can result in physical symptoms such as tachycardia, shortness of breath, dizziness, tremulousness, and difficulty concentrating. Others may experience sleep and gastrointestinal disturbances, headaches or rashes. Children don't like to feel anxious; they are receptive to learning new ways to regain a sense of control. Teaching them relaxation, mental imagery, and biofeedback is an effective strategy. In addition, a child may need psychopharmacologic therapy, counseling, psychodynamic psychotherapy, or cognitive behavioral therapy.

There are children who have specific fears such as a fear of costumes, heights, or bugs. When the fear increases and begins to interfere with everyday functioning, it becomes a phobia. When the child is confronted by the feared object or situation, his coping skills may be overwhelmed, resulting in panic. This process creates a feedback loop that perpetuates the panic.

Often parents assume that their child will outgrow her fear. However, the longer the child's anxiety and fear remain untreated, the more difficult it will be to resolve. The slow exhalation of diaphragmatic breathing stimulates the parasympathetic nervous system. The resulting relaxation response is frequently an integral part of hypnosis. Relaxation can be extraordinarily beneficial, especially when combined with ego-strengthening and desensitization. Visualizing success during hypnosis is a powerful technique to increase feelings of self-efficacy and control.

Habit Disorders

When an action is repeated often enough, it becomes habitual and automatic. The individual performs the behavior with very little, if any, conscious thought. The repetitive act may begin because it provides comfort, or it may result from a physical problem or illness. Some children model their habits after those they see around them. Other habits may result from stress or trauma. Once habituated, the habit may have no relation to the initial trigger.

These repetitive behavior patterns can have serious adverse health effects. They may result in social rejection, teasing, and humiliation. Some children want desperately to stop their habit, but they have no idea how to begin. They may have tried previously, and fear that they will fail again. Other children, for a variety of reasons, have no desire to change. The habit may provide them with comfort or relieve stress. Perhaps the behavior gets them attention and makes them feel special.

For some habit disorders, hypnotherapy may be the primary treatment modality. For others, it can be used as an effective adjunctive therapy. Habits are unconscious, repetitive actions. Therefore, an important first step is developing mindfulness about the behavior. The trance state may be utilized to increase self-control, motivation, and a sense of mastery. In hypnosis, the child can reduce anxiety and imagine a future free from the habit. Ego-strengthening is a vital part of every hypnotic encounter. It reinforces the child's confidence and sense of personal responsibility.

When children learn to control a habituated behavior through hypnotic intervention therapy, it is incredibly empowering. They know that, by tapping into their own inner resources, they have accomplished that feat all by themselves.

Pain

Do you remember when your mother's kiss made a boo-boo all better? Most likely that was the first time you experienced a hypnotic intervention for pain control. Or perhaps it happened when your father tickled your tummy, and you forgot about the headache you used to have.

Pain is a complex phenomenon that can be affected by many factors. Because it is subjective, the experience can be altered. Nowhere is the mind–body–spirit connection so intricately woven as it is when we experience and relinquish pain.

A child who experiences acute pain is already in an altered state of focused attention and highly motivated to seek relief. Anxiety escalates pain, so when working with a child who is anxious and in pain, you must chose your words carefully. "Comfortable," "gently," "soothing," and "easily" replace words such as "painful," "burning," "bad," and "awful." The hypnotherapist's calm confidence can foster positive expectation. Establishing rapport and providing a focus for the child's already intensified attention can reduce fear and anxiety about the pain.

When a child experiences chronic or recurrent pain, he has a sense of negative expectancy. Even when the pain lessens or disappears, he knows it will return. This expectation may result in despair, magnifying anxiety and intensifying the perception of pain.

When children learn during hypnosis the skills that allow them to take charge of their pain, they receive an incredible gift. Hypnosis provides them with active self-management strategies which can restore their sense of self-control and mastery. The techniques may be as simple as distracting a child with fantasy or direct suggestion. A child in pain may be stuck in the kinesthetic mode. Using visual imagery may allow her to see her way to recovery. The skilled hypnotherapist may also use dissociation, distancing from the pain, or focusing attention on it and then changing its size, shape, color, location, or characteristic feel. As with any hypnotic encounter, ego-strengthening suggestions can help the child achieve a measure of success.

Other Uses of Hypnosis

In pediatrics, there are a multitude of clinical applications for hypnosis. The careful use of language and hypnotherapeutic techniques can be incorporated into every pediatric encounter, including health check-ups, visits for acute or chronic illness, hospitalizations, and counseling sessions. Hypnotherapy can be used as an adjunctive therapy for children with psychological disorders such as depression. It can also be helpful for children who have problems with anger management, poor self-esteem, or ADHD. Hypnosis enhances confidence and self-efficacy, allowing the child to focus on a solution rather than the problem.

It is possible to enhance immune function with hypnosis, and thus effectively treat warts. Hypnosis has been used to resolve non-epileptic seizures. Some specialists consider it the definitive therapy for vocal cord dysfunction.

The word "cyber" comes from the Greek, meaning "to steer." Cyberphysiology combines hypnosis and biofeedback. A child can be taught to "steer" his physiology in a beneficial direction. Biofeedback combined with hypnosis can be both fun and instructive for a child, enhancing his sense of mastery and competence. Once he has learned them, he can use these techniques to manage challenges throughout life.

Summary

Metaphorical approaches to problems can bypass resistance by immersing the listener in a fanciful and engaging tale. Older children realize subconsciously the personal relevance of the story. The listener's personal negative internal dialogue may be suppressed, allowing new possibilities to flourish. The goals of these hypnotherapeutic metaphors are altering, reinterpreting and reframing. Most of all, the goal is to ENJOY the magic of imagination.

A Guide to Using the Tales or Tips on Tails

Some of these Harry Tales are entertaining stories with a message that you can read and share with a child. Others, besides being educational and amusing, contain hypnotic scripts and techniques that can be adapted to many different pediatric emotional and physical conditions or problems. Pacing, leading, cadence, rhythm, and vocal inflections are all important in hypnosis. In the scripted portion of the stories, the words to emphasize in a hypnotic intervention are in bold face type.

The story of Harry, Haley, and Conor is a wonderful way to introduce children to hypnosis. Harry is a hippopotamus who has learned hypnotic skills from Dr. Dan, the Ashland Zoo veterinarian. Harry is so good at using his imagination, he is called a hypno-potamus. The hippo helps Haley and Conor learn that when they are feeling sad or angry, they can use their imaginations to think of their favorite things. The tale includes a colorful induction and deepening technique.

Anxiety, Fears, and Phobias

The tales of the hoatzin, octopus, and echidna deal with worries, fears, and anxiety, which are common pediatric problems. The beluga, raccoon, wallaby, and orangutan have more specific fears and phobias. The stork has a difficult time swallowing pills, and the dolphin's anxiety results in selective mutism. Having an invasive medical procedure is the subject of the story of the sea turtle. The story of the loon, and the tale of the hippopotamus and the tortoise, are based on real events that created anxiety in the animals involved.

Fear of Beards *(Page 29)* *(Gabor the Beluga Whale)*

This tale introduces the Ashland Zoo veterinarian, Dr. Dan, who is skilled in the use of hypnosis. Throughout the tales, Dr. Dan helps the animals with their problems by teaching them hypnotic skills.

Fear of costumes, clowns, or masks is not unusual for a young child. Gabor is afraid of masks and beards. Dr. Dan teaches Gabor, a beluga whale, how to tap into his own inner strength to overcome his fear. The tale describes the technique of allowing a child to view what is feared on the television screen of his imagination while he is firmly in control of the remote so he can speed it up, slow it down, or stop the scene entirely. By increments, Gabor gains strength as he moves forward at the speed that is appropriate for him to face his fear. He receives ego-strengthening suggestions as he learns that he is the boss of his fear.

Fear of Trying Something New *(Page 35)* *(Moshe the Happy Hoatzin)*

Moshe, a hoatzin bird from South America, is afraid of leaving the nest and learning to fly. His fears weigh him down. His father places him in the basket of a hot air balloon. The hoatzin's fears and anxieties weigh so heavily on him that the balloon cannot lift upward. Moshe begins to throw some of his fears out of the basket, allowing the balloon to rise to greater heights. Without the fears, Moshe can soar.

Worries and Fears (Page 37) *(Accaria Octopus)*

Accaria Octopus has a lot of worries and fears. This tale contains an induction technique that pairs diaphragmatic breathing with images of waves coming in and going out. Deepening is accomplished by diving down through water. A trunk that Accaria finds at the bottom of the sea is so weighted down with fears that he cannot bring it to the surface. The octopus releases the fears, and the chest becomes lighter, allowing him to bring it to the surface and fill it with courage and confidence instead. Accaria learns that the chest full of strength will always be inside him, available whenever and wherever he needs it.

Post-traumatic Stress Disorder (Page 41) *(Owen and Mzee)*

The tale of Owen and Mzee is based on the true story of an incredible relationship that developed between an ancient tortoise and a traumatized hippo. Owen, the young hippo, has survived a disaster that claimed the lives of his entire family. Mzee, the tortoise, helps Owen to begin having fun again through making art and playing games. The techniques of anchoring and dissociation help the hippo to overcome his PTSD. A soothing, tapping technique helps Owen remember as much of the traumatic event as he wants or needs to. The story also addresses survivor's guilt.

Fear of Bugs (Page 47) *(Bloom Raccoon)*

Bloom Raccoon is afraid of bugs. Dr. Dan helps Bloom by using age regression techniques to bring the raccoon back to before the problem began. Using future progression, Bloom imagines a future that does not include his fear. He learns to be a master gardener in the garden of his imagination.

Invasive Medical Procedure (Page 51) *(Elvira the Green Sea Turtle)*

Having a Voiding Cysto-Urethral Gram (VCUG) can be a frightening and uncomfortable procedure for a child. The tale of Elvira explains having a VCUG. Sea turtles enter a trance state when depositing their eggs, so Elvira learns how to use what she is already good at (dissociation and distraction) and apply it to the new situation.

Selective Mutism (Page 53) *(Meg Dolphin)*

Meg is a bottle-nosed dolphin whose anxiety has caused her to become selectively mute. The dolphin learns diaphragmatic breathing to decrease anxiety. In this metaphor, Meg imagines herself back in a time before the problem began, then she also looks into the future when she is speaking easily. This metaphor also illustrates the forced choice technique: You may … You may … You may … Whatever happens you will … The tale also contains a metaphor about a frog who is trapped in a pit. When his fellow frogs shout to him to give up, the little frog, who is deaf, thinks they are cheering him on, and escapes.

Fear of Heights (Page 59)
(Wester Wallaby)

Wester is a rock wallaby who is afraid of heights. The tale includes an induction technique using both arm levitation and reverse levitation as well as an example of fractionation. Wester also learns how to communicate during a trance by using speech or ideomotor head nodding. The wallaby begins to conquer his fear by learning diaphragmatic breathing in order to calm his whole body and then his heart. The wallaby is able to distance himself from his fear by first watching it on a screen, then seeing his future on the screen free from fear. This tale also incorporates a variation of William Wester's "IT Monster" techniques.

Toileting Anxiety (Page 65)
(Sam Orangutan)

Toileting anxiety is not uncommon in young children. Sam Orangutan is four years old and still in diapers. His interest in trucks inspires a metaphor about a shy pumper fire truck. The fire truck is too shy to use his hose to put out a fire.

When I was working with four-year-old "Lex," who loved trucks, he told me that he thought his penis was too shy, and that's why he couldn't pee anywhere except in his diaper. I mentioned a shy pumper truck who was helped by an older, braver fire truck and suggested that he complete the tale. This bright, creative, and very imaginative youngster created the rest of the metaphor contained in the story of Sam. By doing so, "Lex" resolved his anxiety about toileting. With his permission, and after paying the "fee" of one fire truck, I share his tale with you.

Pill Swallowing (Page 69)
(Irland Stork)

Although children have no problem swallowing a mouthful of food, some children will worry about gagging or choking when swallowing a pill. Irland was afraid to swallow pills. When willpower and imagination are in conflict, imagination always wins. Dr. Dan taught the stork to imagine swallowing easily and comfortably as she had with food in the past. With new confidence the stork practiced first using M&Ms and then successfully mastered the fear that she used to have.

Fear of Change (Page 73)
(Alter Loon)

The tale of Alter the loon is based on the true story of a loon that was rescued from frozen Lake Rescue in Vermont in 2007. The loon was able to change his thinking, alter his perception, and change his behavior. He used his imagination to access pleasant memories and calm himself when he was in stressful situations. Instead of approaching a new situation with dread and fear, Alter learned to view the challenge as an opportunity and an adventure.

Anxiety (Page 77)
(Joe Echidna)

Joe, a very nervous and anxious echidna with a lot of fears and worries, learns to use hypnosis to calm his breathing and imagine that he is in a safe and comfortable place. The narrative describes a deepening technique of not only going down, but also around, in a curly slide. Dr. Dan suggests that worries will not fit down the slide. Many children are very comfortable with computers and competent at using them. Dr. Dan suggests that Joe can drag to the trash, or delete from the computer in his brain, any programs that are not useful—worries and fears, for example. Joe can also download onto his iPod the encouraging and positive things that he needs to hear.

Habit Disorders

Many common habit disorders surface during childhood. Some youngsters may want to stop their habit, but have no idea how to go about it; others think that overcoming it is too difficult. Anxiety often exacerbates the disorder. Hypnotic strategies, combined with relaxation, can be very helpful in helping a child to control a habit. The gibbon's habit of finger sucking provides comfort. The kinkajou's habit cough results from medical problems, then gets stuck. The elephant scratches an itch, then keeps on scratching. Stuttering is a problem for the bonobo.

Habits are things that we can get really good at without giving it much thought. The alpaca is very good at holding back his stool because he remembers that the last time he pooped it hurt. Over time, he holds back his stool automatically, without thinking. Although the quetzal and the vulture have very different problems, similar techniques help them.

Finger Sucking *(Page 81)* *(Gurgevich Gibbon)*

Gurgevich sucks his finger. His dentist uses the Ericksonian technique of prescribing the symptom to help a patient resolve a habit. Becoming mindful of his habit is one of a child's first steps in taking control of his behavior. By assigning a sucking day to each finger, the child becomes mindful, and realizes that he does have control.

Habit Cough *(Page 85)* *(Carol Kinkajou)*

Carol is a kinkajou who develops a habit cough. Dr. Dan teaches her about belly breathing, relaxation, and mental imagery. The story contains a metaphor within a metaphor as Carol remembers a golden fig tree. Little fig tree shoots grow up around the older tree. At first, the shoots develop the habit of growing on and around the tree; then, as the little fig shoots grow and develop strength, the supporting tree no longer serves a purpose, and it quietly dies.

Scratching *(Page 89)* *(Yapko Elephant)*

Yapko Elephant has very itchy skin. Dr. Dan utilizes Yapko's love for video games to create a distraction technique that decreases the elephant's scratching. Yapko also discovers an Itchy Switch that turns down his itching. These techniques empower Yapko to gain control over the scratching.

Stuttering *(Page 91)* *(George Bonobo)*

Anxiety results in George Bonobo's speech dysfluency. Using a yo-yo technique which works well with young children, Dr. Dan teaches the bonobo diaphragmatic breathing. The yo-yo technique allows the clinician to lead and pace a young child until the patient can purposefully belly breathe on his own.

Diaphragmatic breathing is very effective at enhancing relaxation in a child, thus decreasing symptoms that may be exacerbated by anxiety. George visualizes smoothly flowing water. Through imaginary binoculars, the bonobo sees his past before the stuttering began. He also looks ahead to a future without stuttering. Reversing the binoculars, George views the actual time of his stuttering to be quite small and distant. He is able to connect the past with the future so it becomes the present, free of stuttering.

Encopresis *(Page 95)* *(Jud Alpaca)*

Jud Alpaca has a constipation problem that causes encopresis, an emotionally devastating condition for a child. The fecal soiling of encopresis can usually be attributed to overflow incontinence secondary to chronic constipation. The origin frequently dates back to toilet training, and the child's aversion to sitting on the toilet. His desire to avoid the pain of passing a large, hard, constipated stool perpetuates the problem. Because the problem is both physical and psychological, mind–body approaches work best.

This tale explains the problem in a developmentally appropriate way, without blaming the child. It is important for him to learn that he is not the only one in the world with this problem, and that others have successfully learned to be the boss of their poops. Although the child needs to own the problem, his parents must be involved in the initial clean-out, stool softening, and providing a diet rich in fiber, along with plenty of positive reinforcement.

It is child's responsibility to sit on the toilet twice a day. The youngster is also responsible for clean-up and personal hygiene (to the best of his developmental ability). Initially, the child's sphincter has temporarily lost the ability to control defecation, so he should not be penalized for accidents. However, there can be consequences for refusing to sit on the toilet twice a day, or for hiding soiled underwear.

Since success begets success, Jud is encouraged to keep a calendar that rewards even incremental change. In this metaphor, he learns hypnotic techniques to help him relax while taking advantage of the natural gastrocolic reflex during his twice-daily toilet sitting after meals.

Within this tale is another metaphor about a gate keeper who is in charge of opening a gate that lets vehicles pass. The alarm signaling the gatekeeper that a vehicle needs to go through is not working properly. Big tractor trailer trucks cannot pass through without crashing the gate. Meanwhile, small motorcycles, tired of waiting, go around the barrier and sneak right through. Ego-strengthening and visualizing success are important skills to teach any child who has encopresis.

Cyclic Vomiting and Fear of Vomiting *(Page 99)* *(Kluft Turkey Vulture and Kahn Quetzal)*

In the tale of Kluft Turkey Vulture and Kahn Quetzal, Kluft has developed the habit of vomiting, and Kahn is afraid of throwing up. This metaphor explains how to use a chevreul pendulum for determining motivation to change. Although these birds have differing problems, anxiety is a component in both cases, and Kahn and Kluft learn how to resolve it with diaphragmatic breathing and relaxation techniques.

Pain

Some children grow up believing that only medication can reduce pain. They have no idea of the many strategies they can use to increase their comfort. The mongoose has chronically recurring acute pain; the polar bear has acute headache pain; the lion has chronic functional abdominal pain, and the leopard is frequently hospitalized with a serious illness, and experiences iatrogenic pain.

Sickle Cell (Page 105) *(Howard Mongoose)*

Pain is a frequent companion to children with sickle cell. This metaphor illustrates the importance of utilizing what the child brings to the situation. Howard is a pianist. Thus, music is a sensible and effective way to help him manage his pain. The metaphor begins with an eye roll induction. Then, as Howard plays the piano in his imagination, he learns that he can increase or decrease the sound, just like his pain. There is another metaphor within the metaphor about one instrument in an orchestra being out of tune. The conductor asks this instrument to play very softly, until it can be fixed, so the rest of the orchestra can continue to play. The mongoose is able to find his own melody of healing.

Headaches (Page 109) *(Paulker Polar Bear)*

Paulker has a polar bear-sized headache. He imagines the headache as a loaf of bread. The size decreases as he feeds more and more of it to fish. He also discovers that he has a comfort meter that can be turned up. The comfort meter hasn't been working properly. Paulker, however, has in his tool belt all the tools he needs to fix it. Using the words "comforting" and "comfortable" in the metaphor incorporates both the physical and the psychological components of comfort. The polar bear receives several suggestions for decreasing his discomfort: he can take a vacation from his headache, leaving the pain behind, or he can displace it to a part of his body where it will be less bothersome. Since we experience pain only in the kinesthetic mode, visual language takes a child from where he feels bad to where he can see his way to recovery.

Functional Abdominal Pain (Page 113) *(Goldie Lion)*

Goldie Lion has very busy parents—so busy that, at times, Goldie feels forgotten and unimportant. Goldie has developed functional abdominal pain. The metaphor contains an explanation and an example of the mind–body connection that can help children of all ages to understand how their thoughts and worries can affect their bodies.

The tale also contains a metaphor about leaf cutter ants, and how the very tiniest ones, who might seem small and insignificant, are actually very necessary and important. Goldie learns to incorporate all of her senses when she plays the imagination game, and then she uses that ability to comfort and soothe herself.

Hospitalization and Iatrogenic Pain (Page 119) *(Leora Leopard)*

Leora Leopard has been ill with a brain tumor and hospitalized. In this tale, she learns diaphragmatic breathing through bubble-blowing. Bubble-blowing also creates a distraction from painful procedures.

In her imagination, Leora creates a protective bubble that can keep out any hospital unpleasantness. Not only is the bubble filled with comfort and pleasant sensations, it is also a vehicle where Leora can fly away in her imagination to someplace fun, leaving her treatments and the hospital behind.

Other Uses of Hypnosis

The remaining tales are about other uses for hypnosis in pediatrics. From the aardvark tale, the reader can learn hypnotic language and techniques that are useful when examining a young child. The ratel story offers a developmentally appropriate explanation of ADHD and its management. The tale of the platypus introduces biofeedback. Hypnotic techniques help the rhino overcome his vocal cord dysfunction. These skills also help the lizard to get rid of his warts, the panda to overcome non-epileptic seizures, and the horseshoe crab to cope with sleeping problems. The metaphor of the okapi explores the issue of bullies, and the tale of the hermit crab lends itself to a metaphor about being raised in foster care. The hyena is depressed, and the kookaburra is sad and spoiled. The final tale offers some anger management strategies to a kangaroo who throws tantrums, and ends with all the animals in the zoo coming together for a celebration.

Medical Check-up (Page 123)
(Mark Aardvark)

Mark Aardvark is having a medical check-up before entering kindergarten. This tale not only prepares a child for what to expect during a physical examination, it also provides the clinician with hypnotic techniques and language to use with children in a medical setting. The tale includes a strategy for blowing away the pain of an immunization.

Attention Deficit Hyperactivity Disorder (Page 129)
(Raz Ratel)

Raz Ratel has Attention Deficit Hyperactivity Disorder. The story explains ADHD and its pharmacologic management in a manner that is developmentally appropriate for a young child. The tale contains a metaphor within a metaphor as Raz learns about a jeep that has problems with its brakes and steering. An additive in the gas tank helps the jeep to perform much better.

Biofeedback (Page 133)
(Eric Platypus)

Eric the platypus has some worries and some repetitive negative thinking. He learns to calm his body and change his negative thoughts into positive feelings. He uses biofeedback equipment to playfully reinforce the way his thoughts affect his body.

Vocal Cord Dysfunction (Page 135)
(Ran Rhinoceros)

In the tale of the white rhinoceros, Ran has vocal cord dysfunction. His best friend is Mesmer, a bird that eats his ticks and fleas. In the past, scientists thought this was a symbiotic relationship that benefited both rhino and bird. Now it is known that the bird is not such a great friend. It is really after the rhino's blood, and is deliberately delaying wound healing. In the metaphor, the bird pushes Ran into running a race by belittling him. The rhino's stress results in vocal cord dysfunction.

Trance work begins with progressive muscle relaxation that starts at the end of the body that is opposite from the vocal cords, and includes a diaphragmatic breathing exercise. The rhino is reminded that winning and losing is not under his control. The only thing that is under his control is giving his best effort—not because someone else is pushing him to win, but because he wants to run and have fun. The story offers ego-strengthening suggestions along with a reminder about self-serving friendships.

Warts *(Page 139)*
(Lankton Lizard)

Lankton Lizard learns how to effectively stimulate his immune system to eradicate a wart. Like Lankton, children can use visual imagery to imagine their warts being frozen and zapped.

Sleeping Problems *(Page 143)*
(Carolyn Horseshoe Crab)

Carolyn Horseshoe Crab's worries sometimes interfere with sleep. She learns to imagine that she is burying her worries in the sand. The metaphor contains a soothing technique that uses ocean waves and writing sleepy words in the sand. Carolyn times her breathing with the melody of the sea. She pretends that she is sleeping, and then she pretends that she isn't pretending.

Non-epileptic Seizures *(Page 147)*
(Da-Shih Panda)

Psychogenic non-epileptic seizures may be a conversion reaction or a dissociative episode. Rocking motions release endorphins. Da-Shih Panda imagines a rocking motion to self-soothe and enter a trance state. The tale includes the deepening technique of counting backward through descending numbers. The young panda imagines himself grounded, anchored like the roots of a tree, with inner strength that flows through him, allowing him to blossom and flourish. The tale reinforces the importance of regularly practising self-hypnosis.

Depression *(Page 151)*
(Harvey Hyena)

Harvey Hyena is sad and depressed. The zoo psychologist tells Harvey the story of a young hyena that also was sad. An older and wiser hyena advised him to do one thing each day for a week. The tasks included doing something nice for himself, something nice for others, and some physical and mental exercise. Depressed children are often stuck between auditory (hearing negative self-talk) and kinesthetic (feeling down) cues. A therapeutic intervention can allow them to "see." Harvey Hyena begins to look forward to the next day with happy anticipation.

Sad and Spoiled *(Page 155)*
(Burbridge Kookaburra)

Burbridge is a sad and spoiled kookaburra, used to getting whatever he wants, although it doesn't make him happy. There is a metaphor within a metaphor about a cat that is always trying to chase happiness. Under hypnosis, Burbie utilizes his imagination to find a happy, laughing place inside himself. His mood brightens as his selfish, self-centered outlook begins to change.

Foster Care *(Page 159)* *(Maggie Hermit Crab)*

Maggie Hermit Crab has grown up in a number of foster homes. Due to their problems with drugs and alcohol, her parents are unable to care for her appropriately. The metaphor incorporates an induction using a marble. The young hermit crab, confused by her feelings of ambivalence concerning her parents, learns that things can be good, even if they are not perfect. Maggie envisions yelling all her negative feelings into a garbage bag. The hermit crab then uses a side-by-side screen technique, shrinking the bad memories, while enlarging the other screen. This screen reveals what Maggie can do to get herself through a difficult time. This metaphor also incorporates the empowering hypnotic technique of an inner advisor, resulting in increased self-efficacy and self-esteem.

Bullies *(Page 163)* *(Akira Okapi)*

Akira Okapi looks different from the other animals in the zoo and feels that he doesn't fit in. At school, some of the animals bully the okapi. Akira speaks with the principal, who shows him a collection of seashells. Some shells are beautiful on the outside, some on the inside. In his imagination, the okapi travels with the seashell to the bottom of the sea. There Akira passes a school of fish. Some of them are bullying a smaller fish. The little victim learns that bullying is never acceptable. The first thing a bullied fish must do is tell the bullies to stop, that he doesn't like being bullied. Then he must tell an adult and his parents. Once he has done these things, the bullied fish makes a list of all the fish who don't bother him, and circles names of the ones who are nice to him. The fish discovers that he has far more friends than bullies. The metaphor ends with the words of Dr. Seuss: "Be who you are and say what you feel, because those who mind don't matter and those who matter don't mind."

Anger Management *(Page 167)* *(Kenzie Kangaroo)*

Kenzie has a problem controlling her temper. Harry suggests a way for the kangaroo to help herself manage anger. The hippo asks Kenzie to keep track of how many times each day she loses her temper. At the end of the day, the kangaroo punches a tin wall once for each time she has lost control. Soon, the tin wall looks terrible, and Kenzie discovers that it is easier to curb her temper than to keep track of her tantrums and punch the wall.

Harry suggests that for each day that Kenzie controls her temper, she can use a special suction cup to pop out one of the dents in the tin. The kangaroo quickly discovers that repairing the damage her anger has caused takes a long time and a lot of work. Now that Kenzie has learned to control her temper and mend the friendships she lost by throwing tantrums, she decides to give a painting party where all her friends will come to help paint a beautiful picture on the battered tin wall.

All of the Ashland animals are present. They celebrate what they have been able to accomplish by tapping into their own inner strengths by using hypnosis and the power of their imagination.

References

Books and Videotapes

Belnap, Martha. *Taming Your Dragons*. Boulder, CO: The Village Printer, 1986.

Belnap, Martha. *Taming More Dragons*. Boulder, CO: The Village Printer, 1994.

Both books are collections of creative relaxation activities for children. They include breathing exercises, imagery experiences, and playful activities that help children learn skills that help them identify their own moods and understand the importance of self-control and relaxation.

Burns, George. *101 Healing Stories: Using Metaphors in Therapy*. New York: John Wiley & Sons, 2001.
The author is a true artist in the art of storytelling. This book provides the reader with a rich supply of healing stories along with ideas on how to construct meaningful therapeutic metaphors. For each story the author describes the problems it addresses, the resources developed, and what outcomes are offered.

Burton, John, and Bodenhamer, Bob. *Hypnotic Language, Its Structure and Use*. Carmarthen, UK: Crown House Publishing, 2000.
This book is a wonderful resource for beginner clinicians seeking to learn the language of trance, or for experienced clinicians who wish to enhance their language of healing. With strong backgrounds in neurolinguistic programming, the authors provide the reader with insight into the magic of words. They also provide trance scripts and suggest creative methods for inducing cognitive change.

Culbert, Timothy, and Kajander, Rebecca. *Be the Boss of Your Body*. Minneapolis: Free Spirit Publishing, 2007.
This is a series of three books: *Be the boss of Your Stress, Be the Boss of Your Pain*, and *Be the Boss of Your Sleep*. Each volume offers children creative and exciting ways to view the interconnectedness of body, mind, and spirit. These remarkable, kid-friendly books empower youngsters to tap into their own inner resources to help themselves with their problems. Entertaining self-care kits are also available with each book.

Hammond, D. C. (ed.) *Handbook of Hypnotic Suggestions and Metaphors*. New York: W. W. Norton & Co., 1990.
"The big red book," indispensable for anyone who utilizes hypnosis in clinical practice, covers the broad range of uses for hypnosis in medicine, dentistry, and psychology. The contributing authors, who are the best of the best in their field, create a practical, comprehensive desktop reference of "how to" suggestions for clinicians to employ with their patients.

Hilgard, J. R., and LeBaron, S. *Hypnotherapy of Pain in Children with Cancer*. Los Altos, CA: William Kaufman, Inc., (1984).
A comprehensive study of the effects of hypnosis on reducing pain and anxiety in children with cancer. While presenting the results of extensive research, the authors offer developmentally appropriate tools and techniques for both professionals and the parents of children with cancer.

Hunter, Marlene. *Creative Scripts for Hypnotherapy*. New York: Brunner-Routledge, 1994.
A collection of this gifted clinician's favorite hypnotic techniques and approaches, this book is a treasure. Contents include scripts for children to read and use as well as techniques for pain relief, psychosomatic disorders, fears, phobias, habit disorders, and general ego-strengthening approaches.

Klein, Nancy. *Healing Images for Children*. Watertown, WI: Inner Coaching, 2001.
With insight drawn from her personal experience with cancer, the author combines engaging pictures and stories to help children find their own strategies for coping and healing. The book is a wonderful resource for children and their caregivers as they confront cancer or other serious medical conditions. Companion CDs, activity books, and relaxation kits are also available from the author.

Kuttner, Leora. *No Fears, No Tears: Children with Cancer Coping with Pain*. Vancouver, Canada: Canadian Cancer Society, 1986.
Dr. Kuttner is a clinical psychologist who specializes in pediatric pain management. This thirty-minute videotape and manual showcases her work with seriously ill children. The film captures Kuttner's skilled and gentle manner and the effective techniques she employs.

Kuttner, Leora. *A Child in Pain: How to Help, What to Do*. Carmarthen, UK: Crown House Publishing, 2008.
A resource for parents and professionals working with children, this book teaches its readers how to help children of different ages through life's difficult and painful moments.

Kuttner, Leora. *No Fears, No Tears: 13 Years Later*. Vancouver, Canada: Canadian Cancer Society, 1999.
This thirty-minute videotape and manual follows the children who appeared in *No Fears, No Tears* in 1986. Now adolescents and young adults, Kuttner's subjects discuss how hypnosis helped them help themselves, not only with illness, but with life.

Mills, Joyce C., and Crowley, Richard J. *Therapeutic Metaphors for Children and The Child Within*. New York: Brunner/Mazel, 1986.
The authors describe their own applications of Ericksonian approaches to pediatric problems, and provide a framework for understanding the potency of metaphor in blending right and left brain functions. Mills and Crowley also discuss the process of creating therapeutic metaphors to stimulate each person's unique internal resources.

Olness, K., and Kohen, D. P. *Hypnosis and Hypnotherapy with Children* (3rd ed). New York: Guilford Publications, Inc., 1996.
Written by two eminent clinicians, this third edition is a comprehensive guide to pediatric hypnosis, beginning with a historical perspective, and continuing with a review of the literature and its clinical applications. Olness and Kohen provide specific techniques for a variety of pediatric problems, along with examples of actual cases. An indispensable resource for the clinician who works hypnotically with children.

Owen, Nick. *The Magic of Metaphor*. Carmarthen, UK: Crown House Publishing, 2001
The author combines storytelling and metaphor in this collection of seventy-seven stories. The tales promote positive thinking and confidence as they engage and inspire in the search for inner wisdom.

Sugarman, Laurence. *Imaginative Medicine*. Rochester, NY: Pulse Productions, 1997.
Dr. Sugarman, a general pediatrician, created this seventy-minute videotape and learning guide as a practical, in-depth introduction to mind–body methods in pediatrics. The documentary demonstrates hypnotic techniques used daily in a pediatric office, and shows how they comfort children during medical examinations and procedures. The video also shows how hypnotic techniques help children to

manage stress as they cope with chronic illness. Other scenes include personal reports from young people who have utilized self-regulatory strategies to help themselves.

Thomson, Linda. *Harry the Hypno-potamus: Metaphorical Tales for the Treatment of Children*. Carmarthen, UK: Crown House Publishing, 2005.
A collection of thirty-two metaphorical stories that deal with a variety of physical and behavioral problems faced by children. Each tale contains hypnotic language, strategies, and techniques that can be used to empower children and help them with a host of disorders. In addition, there is a section for the clinician explaining how to use the book and the stories it contains.

Wester, William C., and O'Grady, Donald. *Clinical Hypnosis with Children*. New York: Brunner/Mazel, Inc., 1991.
Sixteen experts in the field of hypnosis contributed chapters to this text, which begins with an overview of hypnosis in pediatrics. Subsequent chapters discuss pediatric psychological and medical applications.

Wester, William and Sugarman, Laurence. *Therapeutic Hypnosis with Children and Adolescents*. Carmarthen, UK: Crown House Publishing, 2007.
Compiled in this text are contributions from some outstanding experts in the field of pediatric hypnosis. The first portion of the text provides a broad framework of hypnosis, approaches, and developmental considerations. The latter part of the book focuses on medical and psychological applications of hypnosis with children. Caveats, personal insights, and clinical vignettes enrich this valuable resource.

Zeltzer, Lonnie, and Blackett Schlank, Christina. *Conquering Your Child's Chronic Pain*. New York: Harper Collins, 2005.
Written by two experts in the area of pediatric pain management, this book not only offers accurate information on medical conditions, treatments, and procedures, but also includes advice and practical strategies for ameliorating discomfort.

Information about Hypnosis for Parents

Hypnosis is about learning what you didn't know you knew and controlling what you didn't know you could ... using your mind ... daydreaming on purpose ... thinking to help yourself ... learning how to work to control your mind ...

What is Hypnosis?

Hypnosis is a very old healing modality, a safe, gentle, and effective way to heal, reduce stress, relieve pain, and effect changes in one's life. Hypnosis is a state of mind similar to experiencing a pleasant daydream. People in a hypnotic trance may look like they are asleep, but they are actually relaxed, concentrating, and using their imagination.

If a hypnotherapist is involved, she acts as a coach or facilitator, guiding the person's daydream. The individual patient controls entering and exiting this relaxed state of consciousness. An individual can learn self-hypnosis so he can enter that state of comfort and increased self-control at any time for his own benefit. Learning self-hypnosis is a valuable lifelong skill that is good for the body, mind and spirit.

What is Hypnotherapy?

When a properly trained and credentialed health care professional uses hypnosis as a part of treatment, it is called hypnotherapy. Hypnotherapy is a practical way of helping people manage physical and psychological problems. The hypnotherapist uses relaxation, focused guided imagery, suggestions, and therapeutic metaphors to build self-control over physical and emotional problems.

Contrary to how hypnosis may be portrayed in the movies and on television, the hypnotherapist does not control the individual's behavior. Stage hypnotists take advantage of willing volunteers for the purpose of entertainment. This powerful and personal skill is a gift too valuable for just this purpose. Hypnosis is a state of intense self-control. The therapist may use helpful words to suggest ways to feel, understand, or behave, but she cannot control the person in hypnosis. Although hypnosis makes it easier for people to experience therapeutic suggestions, it does not force them to have these experiences.

All hypnosis is self-hypnosis that can be used for one's own benefit.

What are the Risks of Hypnotherapy?

When used correctly, there are no risks to hypnotherapy, nor any adverse effects. The technique increases one's ability to control symptoms. The brain is incredibly powerful, and contains priceless resources which can be mobilized for personal growth and healing. Hypnosis helps the individual to use his own imagination to tap into his inner strengths and resources. **Hypnosis should only be used as part of a treatment plan for a specific problem after a careful evaluation by a trained health professional.**

Why Use Hypnotherapy?

Hypnotherapy has been used successfully to treat pain, anxiety, fears, phobias, pain, asthma, bedwetting, stool-withholding, nervous tics, smoking, obesity, and many other problems. **The value of hypnosis goes beyond its ability to help with these ailments**. Increasing one's ability to control symptoms through hypnosis can strengthen confidence and mastery. Personal success in self-hypnosis increases self-esteem. Self-hypnosis is a skill that increases with practice. The techniques can be used to meet new challenges throughout life.

For more information about the use of hypnosis with children contact:

American Society of Clinical Hypnosis
140 N. Bloomingdale Road
Bloomingdale, IL 60108-1017
www.asch.net
Phone: 630-980-4740
Fax: 630-351-8490
Email: info@asch.net

Society for Developmental and Behavioral Pediatrics
6728 Old McLean Village Drive
McLean, VA 22101
www.sdbp.org
Phone: 703-556-9222
Fax: 703-556-8729
Email: info@sdbp.org

The Tales for Children

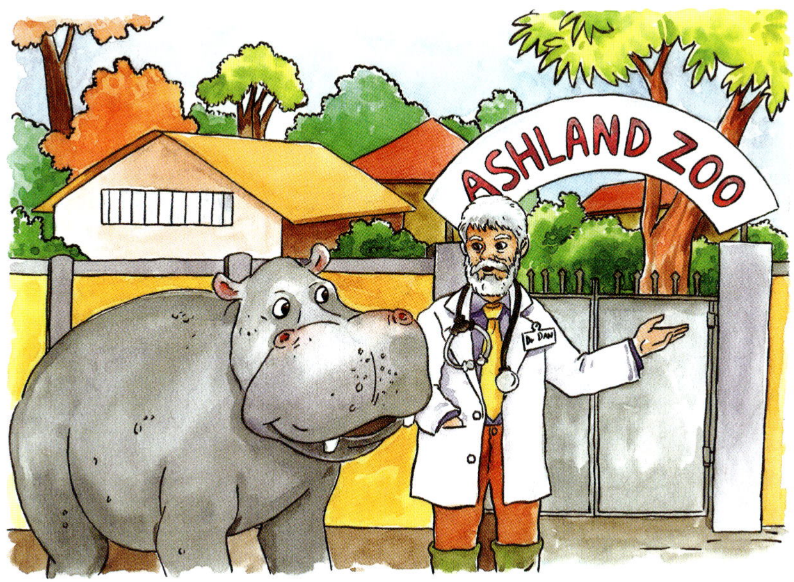

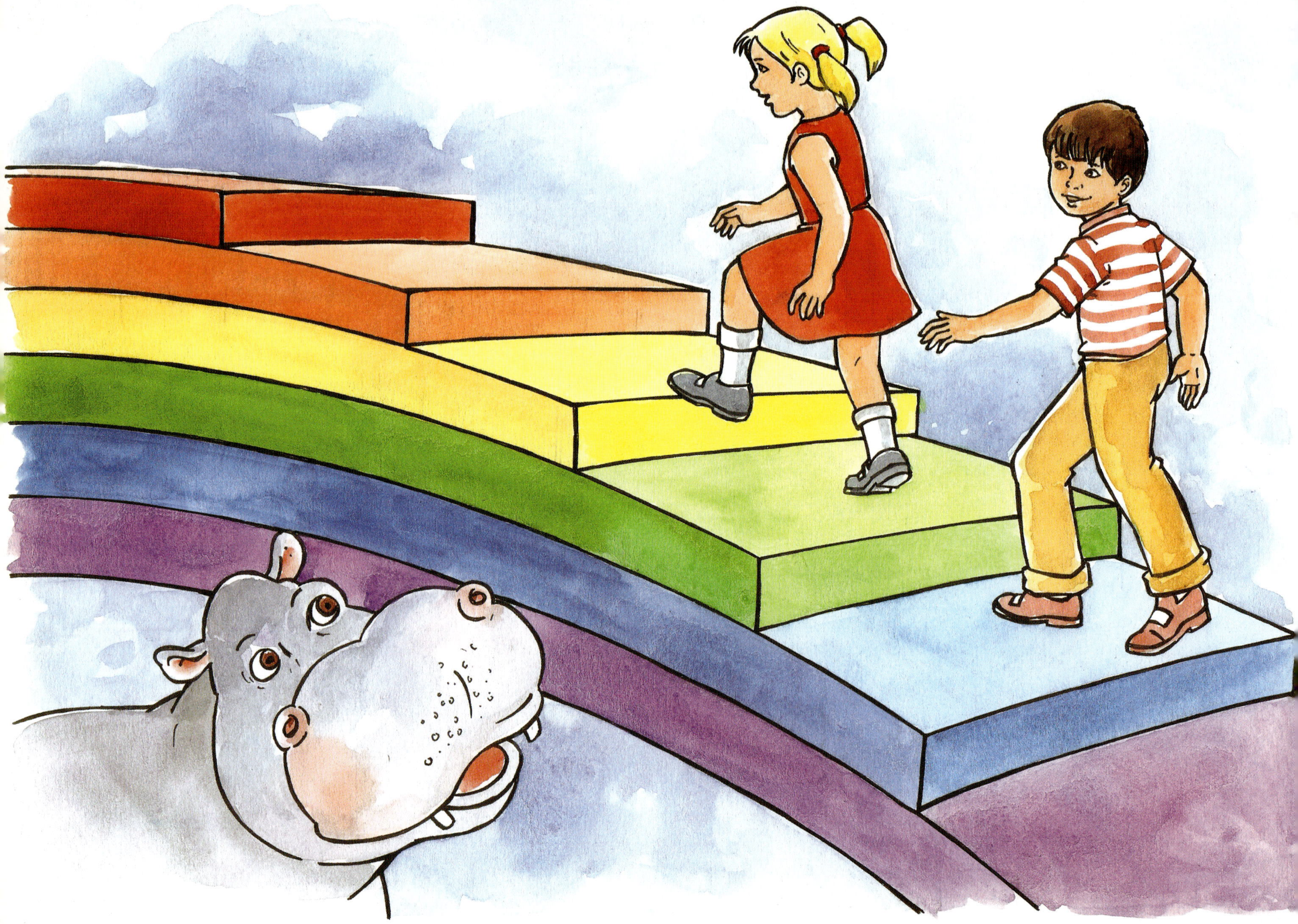

Harry Teaches Haley and Conor About Hypnosis

Harry is a hippopotamus who lives at the Ashland Zoo. His favorite place at the zoo is a big mud puddle where he loves to splash around and duck under the water and pretend he is a submarine.

Harry has a wonderful imagination. His friends at the zoo call him Harry Hypno-potamus because he is so good at using his imagination to help himself when he is feeling scared or sick.

One morning, as Harry splashed happily in his mud puddle, he heard a little girl singing. Pretty soon, Harry's friend, Haley, and her cousin, Conor, skipped through the zoo's stone gate. They came to the zoo often. Haley, Conor, and Harry were good friends.

Harry popped up from the mud puddle with a toothy grin. "Haley!" he cried, "was that you singing?"

Haley nodded her head up and down so her long blond pigtails bounced on her shoulders.

"Yes, it was," she said.

Harry settled back in his mud puddle to listen to Haley singing. It was a song about a rainbow.

"What a wonderful song!" said Harry.

"I love rainbows," Haley told him. "Would you like to hear another song?"

"I sure would!" Harry answered, blowing happy bubbles in the mud.

Haley rose up on her tiptoes and sang in a high, clear voice, about all the things she liked best. Conor joined in too. Thinking and singing about special things helped when they were sad or feeling bad.

"Wow!" Harry exclaimed. "That's just like hypnosis! When I feel worried or sad or sort of yucky, I think of my favorite things and then I don't feel so bad."

"What's hypnosis?" Conor asked.

"Well," said Harry, "it's a special kind of thinking you can do to help yourself. I already sort of knew how to do hypnosis, but I didn't know what it was called. It is like daydreaming, or pretending on purpose. It's like thinking to help yourself. Dr. Dan, the zoo's veterinarian, taught me how to do it. It's fun, and you can use it for all kinds of things."

"What sort of things?" Haley asked.

"Well," said Harry, "my friend Brownie, the bat, had trouble sleeping. Dr. Dan taught Brownie hypnosis to help him sleep. Mitch Monkey used his imagination to help himself play basketball better. Another friend, Molly Macaw, had this bad habit of pulling out her feathers. After a while, she had hardly any feathers left. Dr. Dan taught her how to use hypnosis so she could get over that habit she used to have. Now she has the most beautiful feathers in the zoo! Pam Penguin used hypnosis and her imagination when she had an operation. It helped her to get better faster."

"It sounds like magic," Haley said.

"Imagination does work like magic," Harry replied. "Once, when I had a very bad toothache, I used my imagination to pretend I was in Africa in a giant mud puddle. I got so busy thinking about that mud puddle that I didn't think about my toothache anymore."

Harry stood up and let the mud slide off his thick, gray hide, then he sat down beside Haley and Conor.

"Hypnosis is really fun. I like to practise even when I don't have any problems. The more I practise, the better I get at using my imagination. It is like a present I can give to myself every day."

"Could you teach us?" Haley asked.

"Of course," Harry replied. "First, get nice and comfortable. You can close your eyes or keep them open, whatever you would like or want to do … now. That is the best part about hypnosis: there is no wrong way to do it, whatever works best for you, because you are in charge of your imagination. You are the boss of your pretending.

"Since you like rainbows, perhaps you would like to imagine a big beautiful rainbow. Just like in your song, we could go over the rainbow. There are steps going up the rainbow. Each step to the top of the rainbow is a different color.

"One. The first step is red. As you stand on the red step, think of one of your favorite things that is the color red—perhaps a beautiful red sunset, or maybe a big red balloon, or a shiny red apple.

"Two. The next step is orange. I wonder what favorite thing you will think of that is orange.

"Three. Then comes yellow. I know what my favorite thing is that is the color yellow, but yours may be different—whatever you want it to be.

"Four. The fourth step is green. Imagine something green that you really like.

"Five. Blue is the color of the next step."

"This is fun!" said Conor. "I am pretending I am riding my new blue bicycle."

"Six. The last step at the top of the rainbow is purple."

"Oh goodie!" said Haley "That's my favorite color."

"Those six steps take you to the top of the rainbow, and now you can choose how you want to go **down** the other side of the rainbow in your imagination. You could ride a bike **down**, or maybe slide **down** on a sled, or find another fun way. Whatever your imagination wants to do to take you over the rainbow, where troubles melt like lemon drops, where nothing needs to make you sad or worried, where tummy aches or boo-boos don't need to bother you because you are having fun. You are the boss of your imagination. You are pretending on purpose. You are in charge.

"Your imagination lives inside your brain, so it is always there for you to use whenever and wherever you need or want to use it. The more you practise hypnosis, the better you get at it."

"That was really cool!" Haley said.

"I loved using hypnosis," said Conor. "It made my whole body feel good, relaxed, and comfortable. I am going to practise every night at bedtime."

"That's wonderful!" Harry replied. "You could be Conor Hypno and maybe Hayley could be the Imagination Princess!"

Gabor the Beluga Whale

It was October, and all of the animals at the Ashland Zoo were getting excited about Halloween. Halloween is the day when everybody at the zoo dresses up in a costume and mask and pretends to be a princess or a super hero, or even a different animal or bird. There would be a parade and prizes for the best disguise. The animals would try to guess who was really behind each mask.

Harry decided to wear a horn on the tip of his nose. "That'll make me look a lot like Ran Rhino," he said to himself.

Akira Okapi, whose back side already had stripes, decided to paint black lines on the rest of his body so he would look like a zebra. Dr. Dan already had white hair and a white moustache, so he thought he would dress up for Halloween with a long white fake beard.

Gabor was a beluga whale. Before he came to the Ashland Zoo, he had lived in the Arctic Ocean. When Gabor was born, his skin was a brownish-blue color. Now that he was five years old, he was white. Belugas are called "sea canaries" because their songs and chatter can be heard above the water even when they dive deep under the ice. These whales are very sociable, and they like to live together in groups called pods.

Belugas love parties, and so did Gabor. However, he hated Halloween.

"Why?" asked Gabor's good friend, Harry Hypnopotamus, who loved dressing up and pretending.

"It's the clowns and masks and disguises. They scare me," Gabor said. "Trick or treating sounds like fun, but everybody dresses up in costumes."

"Why don't we swim over and see Dr. Dan," Harry suggested. "He can help you be the boss of your imagination and your fear."

Dr. Dan was the vet who took care of all the animals at the Ashland Zoo. Everybody loved him. Not only did he give the animals their check-ups and take care of them when they were sick, but he knew all about hypnosis. He liked to share those skills with his animal friends.

"You have very special abilities inside your brains," Dr. Dan told them. "Maybe you never even knew they were there. Learning how to do hypnosis can help when you are worried or afraid."

When someone had a habit that got in the way of having fun—wetting the bed, for example—Dr. Dan helped them with hypnosis. He even taught some of the animals who were uncomfortable and in pain how to decrease their discomfort and increase their comfort by tapping into special skills inside their own brains. Harry the hippopotamus was especially good at using hypnosis. That's why he was called Harry Hypno-potamus.

Gabor waggled his flippers with excitement. "Let's go see him right now!" he said.

The two friends arrived at Dr. Dan's office just as he was trying on his costume for the Halloween parade. Gabor took one look at Dr. Dan with his long white beard, and he got very scared. He started to cry. Right away, Dr. Dan took off the beard and began speaking gently with Gabor about his fears.

"Would you like to learn to be the boss of your fears?" he asked Gabor.

"I sure would!" Gabor said. "I'm tired of missing out on fun stuff because I get scared."

"Imagine that you are diving deep **down** into the ocean," said Dr. Dan, "going down **deeper** and **deeper**, getting **more** and more **relaxed** the **deeper** you go."

As Gabor went deeper and deeper he noticed, in his imagination, all the beautiful colored fish, the coral sea fans, and the sea grass waving gently back and forth. Using his imagination to think about something fun made Gabor feel calm and relaxed.

While Gabor was feeling safe and nicely relaxed, Dr. Dan asked him to picture, on the TV screen of his imagination, his friend Harry the Hypno-potamus getting ready for the Halloween parade.

"He is putting a big horn on top of his head, pretending to be a rhino," said Dr. Dan. "Remember," he told Gabor, "you control the remote for the TV of your imagination. If you begin to feel afraid, you can stop it and rewind. You can tell yourself, 'Fear, I am stronger than you are. You are not getting the best of me. I am stronger than you are.'"

Then Dr. Dan suggested, "When you are ready, feeling **calm** and **strong**, you can push the play button on the remote control of your imagination. Your remote is a very special one. It can zoom in close, or it can zoom out so you can watch the animals getting into their Halloween costumes from a safe distance away.

"Then, not before you are ready—now—to breathe in that **confidence** ... and let go of doubts, ... breathe in **strength** ... and let go of fears, as you zoom in a little closer. Stop anytime you want or need to, gather strength, noticing how **calm** and **comfortable**, **confident** and **in control** you are as you continue to go forward in the direction you wish to go—slowly at first, and then faster as you gather **strength** and **confidence**. Hear yourself say, 'I can do this. Fear is just a thought in my imagination, and **I am the boss** of my imagination. **I am the boss** of my fear.'"

Gabor breathed in strength and breathed out his fear. In his imagination he watched the Halloween parade at the zoo. He realized that there was nothing about the masks or face paint to be afraid of. The animals were all his friends. Putting on a mask was like putting on a mitten or a shoe. It didn't change who you were.

Dr. Dan suggested, "Come back up from the bottom of the sea of your imagination and bring back with you all that strength and **confidence**, that '**can do**' attitude. It would be all right to leave the fear behind, coming up through the water, ... more and more alert, ... feeling good, ... **feeling proud**, ... **the boss** of your imagination, and **the boss** of the old fear you used to have."

"Wow!" said Gabor. "Hypnosis is really cool!"

"Would you would like to stay and help me get ready for the Halloween parade?" Dr. Dan asked the beluga whale.

"Yes," Gabor said.

The beluga rose up on his tail and helped Dr. Dan fasten a long white beard on his chin. With his flippers, Gabor helped Dr. Dan tug on his big clown feet. Next came a silly coat that made Harry giggle. Finally, they all went to the Halloween parade.

When the three friends got there, all the animals shouted, "Hey, Ran Rhino, you forgot to dress up!"

They were surprised to discover that Ran was really Harry wearing a rhino horn.

Carol Kinkajou covered parts of her brown fur with the white pollen of the balsa flower so she looked like a baby panda. Carol's cousin, Bloom, the racoon, having conquered his fear of bugs, came dressed as a

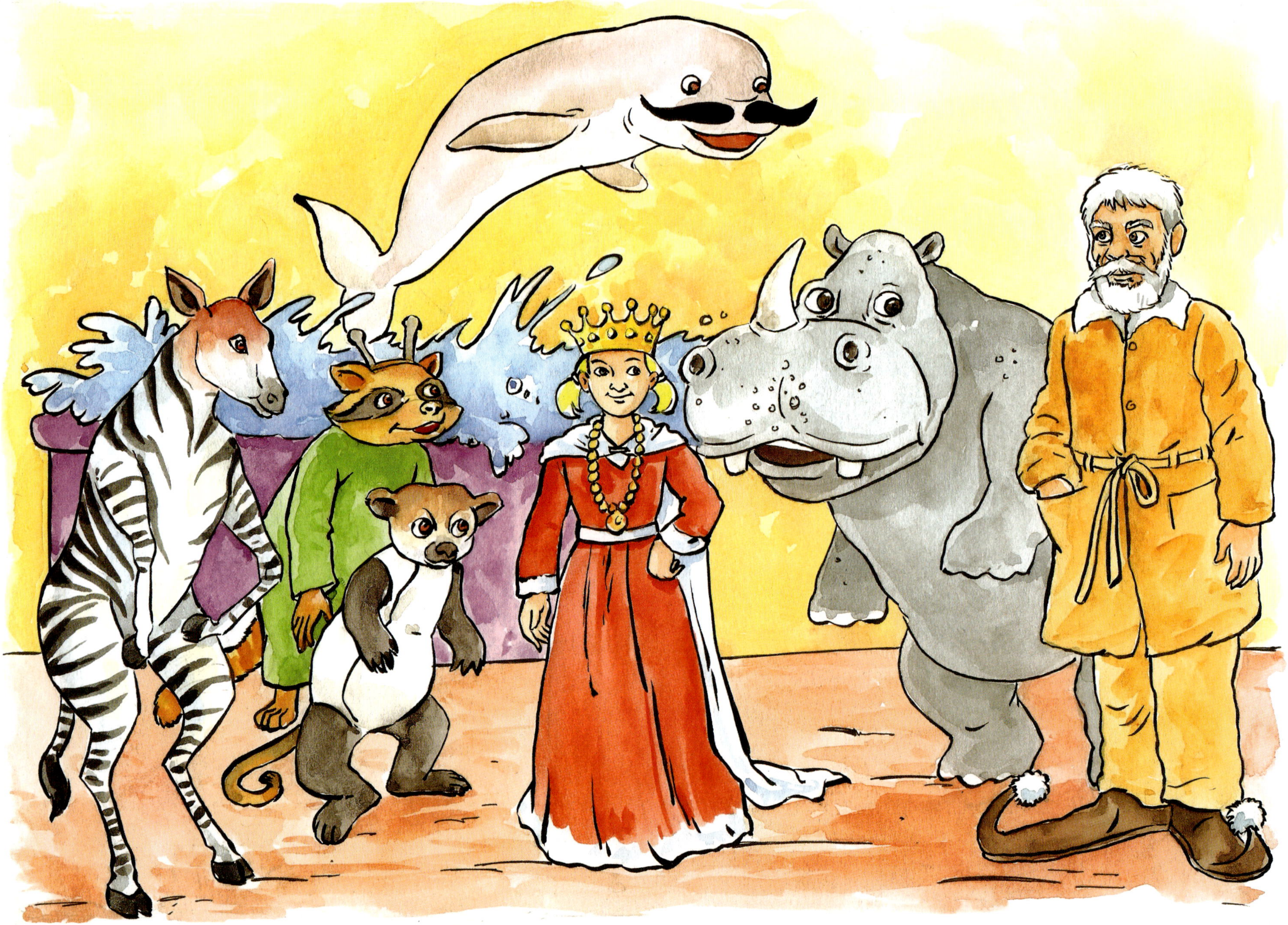

beetle. Harry's friend Haley was a beautiful princess. Everyone loved Dr. Dan's clown costume and long white beard the best. They all agreed that he looked very distinguished with a beard.

"You should grow one," Haley said.

Dr. Dan thought a moment. "I'll do just that."

Watching the parade, Gabor felt good. "I'm not scared at all," he told Dr. Dan. Then he surprised himself as he said, "I think I would like to dress up too. I have always liked Tom Walrus's big mustache."

"I have just the thing," Dr. Dan replied. He snipped a piece of fur from his long, white beard, then borrowed some ink from Accaria Octopus so he could dye the fur black. Finally, he made a great big black moustache for Gabor, and together they joined the parade.

Dr. Dan walked along beside the whale, who was floating in a big tub of water pulled by Harry Hypnopotamus and Yapko Elephant. After the parade, they all went trick or treating. It was so much fun! Gabor had such a big smile on his face that even the ends of his moustache curled up in a great big grin.

"I'm the boss of my fear!" he shouted, and he clapped his flippers.

So that is how Dr. Dan came to grow a beard, and how Gabor overcame his fear of clowns and beards and masks.

Sometimes, even when it isn't Halloween, Gabor dresses up with a moustache that always seems to curl up in a big beluga grin.

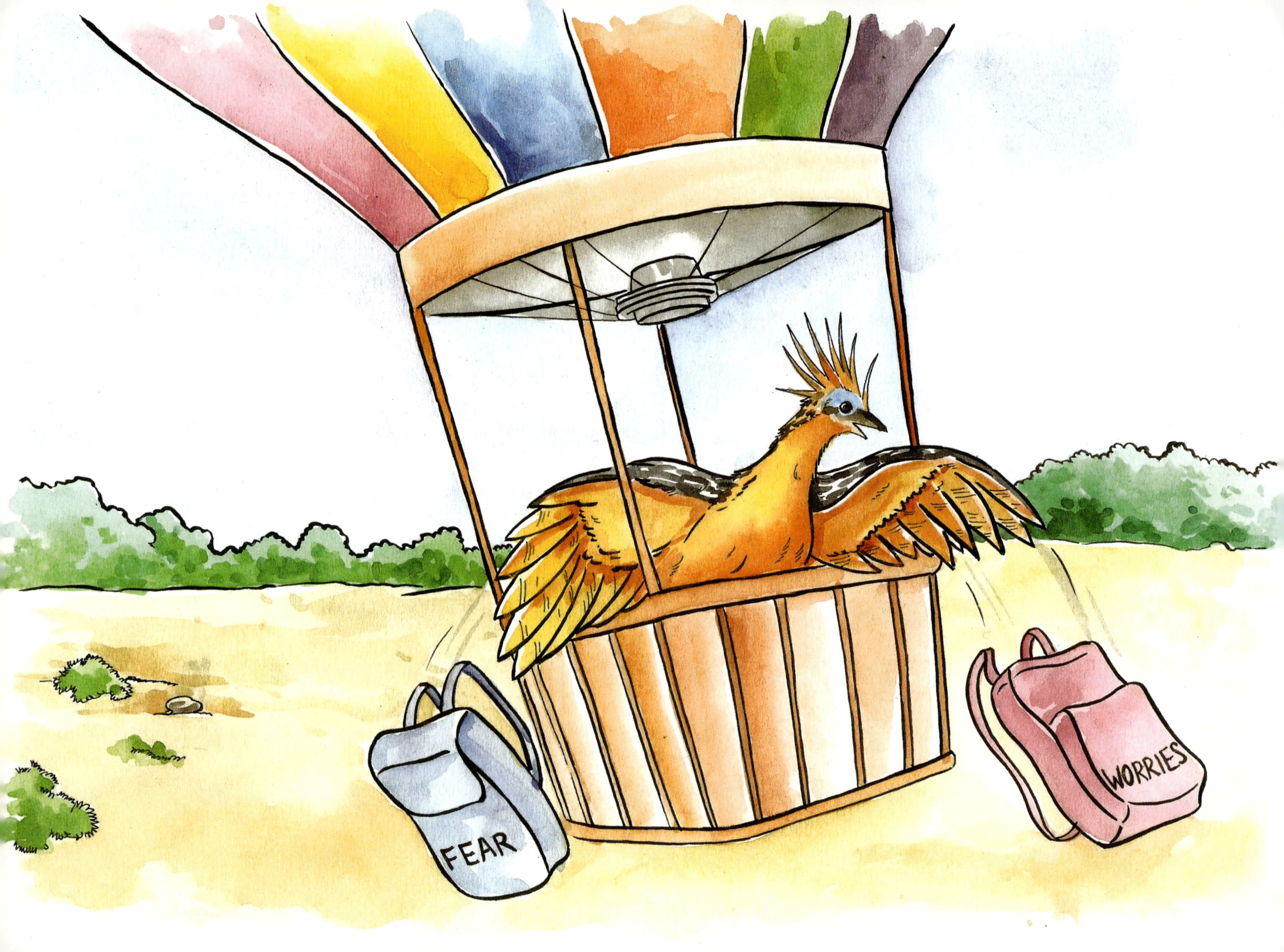
FEAR
WORRIES

Moshe the Happy Hoatzin

Moshe was a hoatzin bird. He came from the Amazon River in Peru. When he arrived at the Ashland Zoo, Moshe met Harry the Hypno-potamus and they became good friends.

Hoatzin birds have been around for thousands of years. The mother lays her eggs in a nest on a tree branch that reaches out over the water of a stream below. When Moshe and his brothers and sisters were just baby birds, and too young to fly, their mother would push them out of the nest if she thought they were in danger. The babies would fall down into the water below.

Unlike any other bird, hoatzin babies have special claws on their wings that allow them to climb up a tree and back to their nest when danger has passed.

Moshe told Harry, "When I was a baby bird, I hated it when my mother pushed me out of the nest, even though I knew she was trying to protect me. I didn't like the drop down into the water; it scared me. The climb back up was pretty scary, too.

"Just like a tadpole who loses his tail when he turns into a frog, I lost my special claw as I got older. Without that claw to help me climb back into my nest, I needed to learn how to fly. I didn't want to learn to fly. I wondered why I couldn't just stay in the nest. I liked it there.

"My brothers and sisters couldn't wait to learn. Very soon, they were flying around the treetops. I was worried about failing, falling, and not having claws to climb back up to my nest. Those worries weighed me down. When my mother gently nudged me from the nest for my first flight lesson, my muscles were so tight I couldn't make my wings work right. I was so weighed down with worry, I fell straight down to the ground."

Harry said, "I've noticed how good you are at flying around the zoo. How did you get from being on the ground, and so afraid that you wouldn't even try to fly, to soaring through the treetops the way you do now?"

The hoatzin told Harry, "I had a very wise father. Very gently, he placed me in a tiny basket. Then he attached a brightly-colored helium balloon to the basket. Helium balloons, you know, are filled with a special kind of air that makes them lift up into the sky.

"My father said that the helium balloon would lift me and my basket back to my nest. Well, that didn't happen. All my worries and fears made the basket so heavy, the balloon couldn't lift up.

"Unless I got rid of my fear, I would be stuck on the ground, and I'd miss out on all the fun my brothers and sisters were having. Finally, I decided to let go of a little of my fear. I dropped it over the side of the basket. As soon as I did that, the basket began to lift a little bit. I tossed some worries out of the other side of the basket, and the bright helium balloon lifted me a little bit more.

"I discovered that getting rid of worries was a lot more fun than being weighed down by them. Not only did the balloon lift higher, so did my spirits. I discovered that I liked being up in the air. As the basket went higher and higher, I felt lighter and lighter, and more and more free.

"Soon, without the weight of my worries holding me down, I was all the way up to my nest high in the treetops. I told my dad, 'Now I feel free, and light enough to fly. I feel ready and confident, and powerful and strong.'

"I realized that I didn't miss any of my old worries. Those old silly fears, and being afraid to try, had almost caused me to miss flying."

"That's a great story," Harry said. "I liked hearing about how you got to be the boss of your fear, and learned to control what you never knew you could."

Moshe told Harry the Hypno-potamus, "Being free of my worries, and being free to fly, makes me a very happy hoatzin."

Accaria Octopus

Accaria Octopus lived in the ocean. He had a large head, big eyes, and eight long arms. If Accaria sensed danger, or a predator threatened him, he had a lot of great ways to escape. First, he would try to hide in plain sight. His skin would change color so the octopus could blend in with the colors, patterns, and textures around him.

Sometimes, in spite of the camouflage, a predator might spot Accaria. When that happened, the octopus could squirt out ink that made the water so dark the predator couldn't see him escape. Accaria was a very fast swimmer. While he was getting away, the ink went up the predator's nose so he wouldn't be able to smell where the octopus was hiding.

Accaria was very good at finding hiding places. He could squeeze his rubbery body into very small cracks and crevices. If a predator did come after him, the octopus would paralyze his enemy with a poisonous bite. If a big predator grabbed hold of one of the octopus's eight arms and pulled it off, Accaria could grow a new one.

Although the octopus was very clever at avoiding danger, being chased all the time is scary, and Accaria had a lot of fears and worries. The other animals sometimes teased him and called him "Accaria Scared-ee-a."

One day, as the octopus lay on a rock beside the ocean, he told his friend, Harry Hypno-potamus, about his fears. Harry never liked to tease anyone.

"I used to have a lot of fears, too," Harry replied. "Then Dr. Dan taught me how to help myself with hypnosis."

"Who is Dr. Dan?" asked Accaria.

"He's the vet at the Ashland Zoo where I live," Harry replied.

Although Harry was too modest to say so, he had gotten to be so good at using hypnosis that everybody called him "Harry the Hypno-potamus.

"You could talk to Dr. Dan about your fears and worries," Harry suggested.

The next morning, Dr. Dan came down to the seashore.

"Accaria," he said quietly.

As soon as he heard the vet's voice, Accaria eased himself out of the cave where he had been hiding. Slowly, arm over arm, he crept to the shore.

"Harry tells me that you would like to learn to use your imagination on purpose to help yourself with your worries," said Dr. Dan.

Accaria nodded his big, round head. "Sometimes my fears and worries get in the way of fun stuff," he said.

"Why don't you get comfortable," Dr. Dan suggested. "Now, breathe in as you imagine a wave coming into the shore … As you let go of your breath, the wave will go back out to sea … As you breathe in, the wave comes in, … and as you breathe out, the wave goes out, taking you **deeper** and **deeper relaxed**, breathing in … and out with the waves, … going **deeper** … and **deeper** relaxed.

"Now, imagine that you are diving **down** deep into the ocean. The **deeper** you swim, … the more **relaxed** you become … **Deeper** and **deeper**. When you arrive at the bottom of the sea, imagine a big trunk or chest. The chest is filled with all your worries and fears. The worries and fears make the trunk so heavy that even with all eight arms you are having trouble bringing the chest up to the surface. Your worries weigh the trunk down too much. Perhaps you would like to let some of your worries go."

As Accaria let the worries go, the chest became lighter and lighter, and he was able to swim with it all the way to the surface.

As Accaria took the chest to the shore, Dr. Dan said, "It would be fun to fill the now empty chest with good feelings. In your imagination, look for seashells, noticing that each sea shell is labeled something different. There is one labeled 'Courage,' another 'Pride.' There is a beautiful shiny shell labeled 'Strength,' and a large one labeled 'Self-esteem.' "

Accaria found a great shell that was "Bravery." Since he had eight arms, he was very good at gathering up all the good-feeling shells and filling the chest full. It was so full of good stuff, there was no room for worries.

Now Accaria could take the chest, which was inside his imagination so that it would always be with him, back to the bottom of the sea where he lived. All those

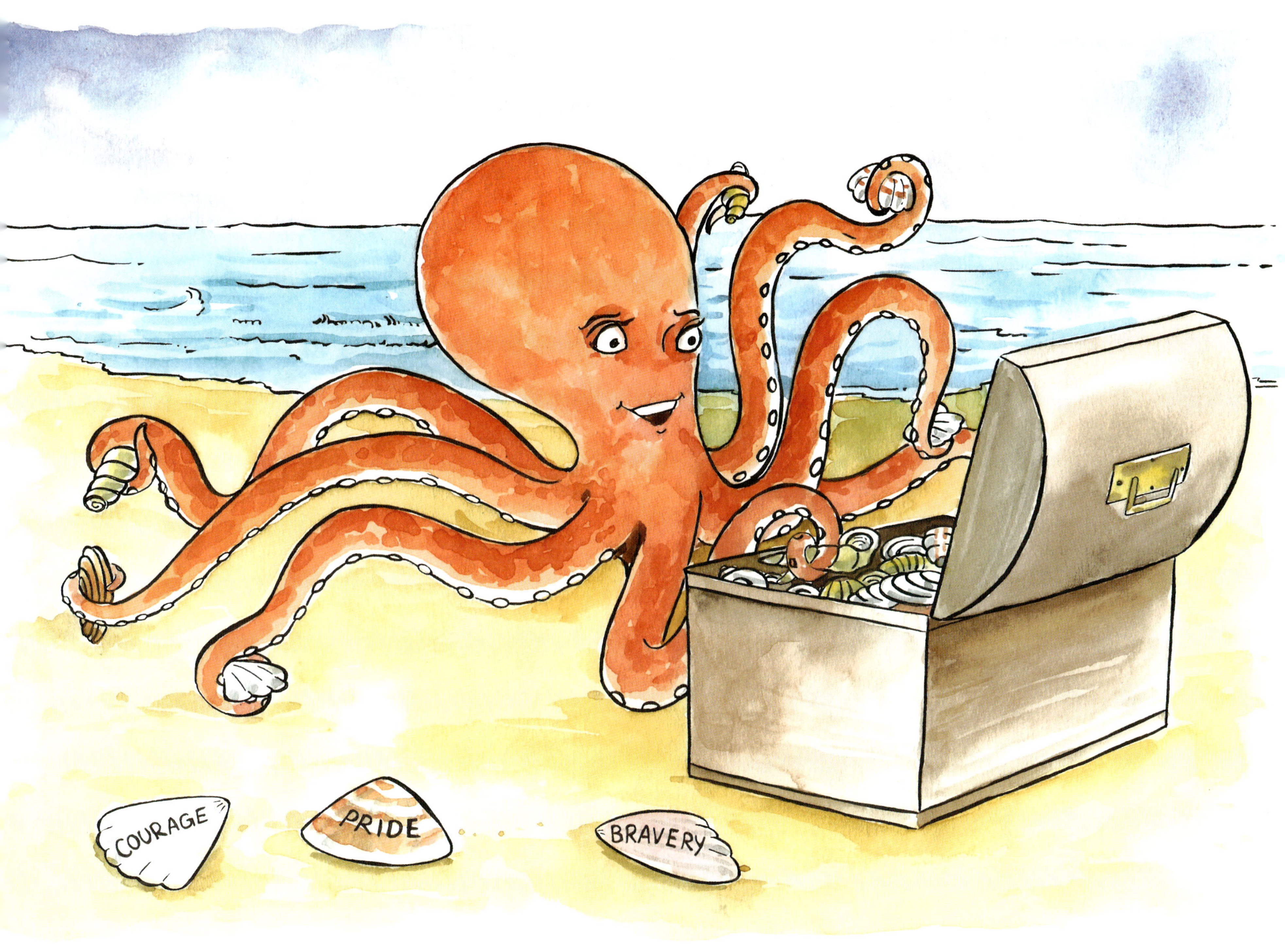
COURAGE
PRIDE
BRAVERY

good feelings were right there with him replacing the old worries he used to have.

"Whenever you are finished with your hypnosis, your imaginings," suggested Dr. Dan, "you can just pretend to swim up from the bottom of the sea, bringing back with you all that courage, all those good feelings that are now part of you. No one will ever call you 'Accaria, the Scared-ee-a' again."

And nobody ever did.

Owen and Mzee

This tale is based on the true story of a friendship between a young baby hippo and a giant ancient tortoise. It happened in Kenya, Africa at the time of the great tidal wave in December 2004.

A baby hippopotamus, not yet one year old, lived with his hippo family in Kenya. The hippos enjoyed wading out into the muddy Sabaki River.

One day, heavy rains came. The river flooded, washing the hippos out to sea. Then, an earthquake at the bottom of the Indian Ocean caused a giant wave, called a tsunami, to rise up out of the sea. This huge wall of water spread out in all directions, flooding the land and sweeping away buildings, humans, and animals. The hippo family drowned in the giant wave. Only the baby survived.

The baby hippo was washed up onto a shelf of land near the shore. He was exhausted, confused, and terrified. The villagers who had survived the tsunami saw the little hippo on the sand bar and set out to rescue him. They captured the hippo and loaded him onto a truck.

The hippo had never seen humans before. The truck was noisy, and the ride was bumpy. The hippo baby was scared, and he felt all alone. The men named the hippo "Owen," after the man who had gone out to the sand bar to save him. They took Owen to a nature reserve near Mombasa. When they got the hippo off the truck, he ran and hid behind a rock where he began to cry. Big hippo tears ran down his cheeks. Owen had been washed away from his home, and all of his friends and family were gone. The baby hippo was alone in a strange place without any friends.

Suddenly, the rock moved and began to talk.

"Don't cry, little hippo," the rock said. "I'll be your friend."

The rock was actually a giant tortoise named Mzee who was more than 130 years old. He became Owen's very first friend. A hippo usually stays with its mother for four years, so Owen pretended that Mzee was his mother. When it was time to sleep, Owen lay down next to Mzee, rested his head on the tortoise's shoulder, and cried.

One of the workers at the nature reserve told Mzee the story of how Owen came to live there.

"After a terrible storm," he said, "all of Owen's family got washed out to sea. Then a tsunami came and drowned all of Owen's family. The baby hippo was the only one who survived. Some strangers caught Owen and put him in a truck. They brought Owen here, to this place where he has never been, and where he doesn't know anybody.

"No wonder he is so sad, and cries so much," the tortoise said.

Tortoises are very good at looking like a rock. They don't move very much or very fast. That suited Owen just fine; he didn't feel like moving, or playing, or having any fun.

Mzee was very old and very wise. He knew that it was important for the young hippo to begin to play again, and to smile, and have fun. They began to walk around the nature reserve together. Mzee found a ball and they began to kick it back and forth. Mzee got some crayons for Owen so he could color and draw, or write about his feelings.

Mzee knew that hippos are supposed to love the water. In fact, the word "hippopotamus" means "water horse." However, any time that Owen got near the water, or if it began to rain, the hippo would start to panic. His heart would beat really fast. He felt like he might throw up, and it became hard for him to breathe. His body would start to shake.

Owen didn't know why he felt like this. He didn't remember what had happened to him. His inside brain remembered that it was something bad, and it had to do with water.

Mzee remembered the story of what happened to Owen, and how he came to live at the nature reserve. He knew why, every time they walked close to the water in the pond, Owen stopped, and got panicky and scared.

Mzee stopped and lay down in the grass. Owen lay down next to him, resting his head on Mzee's front leg. Owen felt safe and secure next to Mzee. He watched the fluffy white clouds floating across the blue African sky. All of Owen's muscles felt relaxed and comfortable.

Mzee suggested, "Remember the taste of your favorite food … Mmmmmmm … Breathe in the smell of the grass … Perhaps you would like to feel yourself gently rocking in a hammock … **safe** and **comfortable** …

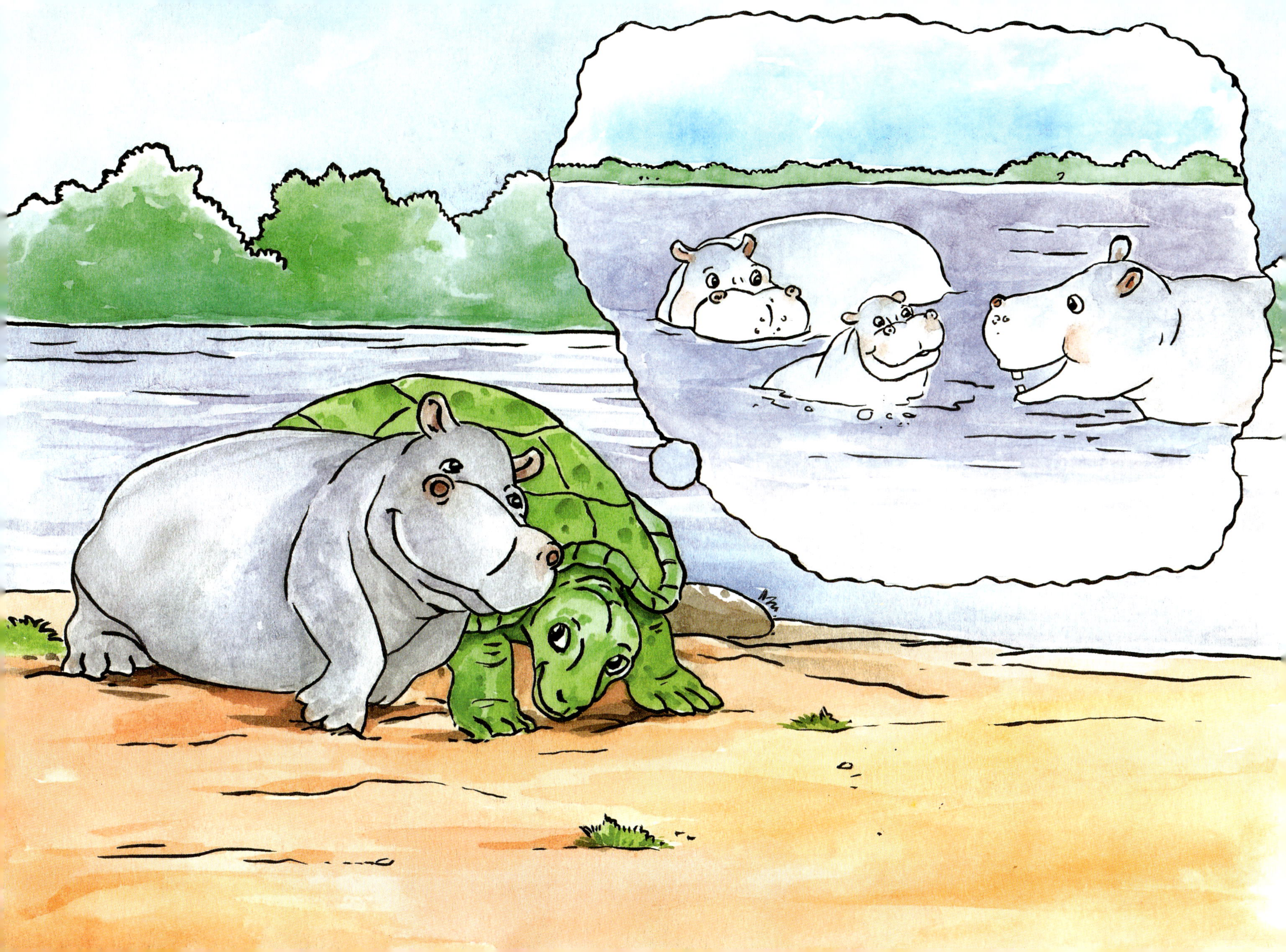

gently back and forth. Hear the wind moving the branches in the trees … feel the gentle breeze on your face … and how **good** the warm sun feels on your back.

"Imagine yourself in a favorite place, on a very special day, feeling good, relaxed and **comfortable** … That's right."

Mzee asked Owen, "Where are you, in your imagination?"

Owen said, "I am with my family, near the Sabaki River."

Mzee said, "Isn't it interesting that you can be here with me, completely **safe** and comfortable, feeling the ground beneath you, while in your imagination, you are back with your family near the Sabaki River. Would it be all right, while you are here, feeling **safe** and **secure**, to go closer to the river in your imagination?"

Owen let his head nod, "Yes."

"As you get closer to the water, in your imagination, cross your arms across your chest, and tap **gently** with the rhythm of your mother's heart beat. That's right, gently tapping as you go into the river with your family. Continue tapping as the clouds move in, and it begins to rain, and the river rises, remembering as much, or as little, as you want or need to, all the while knowing that you are here, **safe** and **comfortable**, as you gently continue tapping.

"You may choose to fast forward at any time, on the screen of your imagination, because you are the boss of your imagination. You are **in control**. Know that you were able to accomplish something amazing. You survived. You are here now, tapping gently.

"Sometimes, wounds that are covered up don't heal. Taking all the time you need … **Healing** … **Mending** … Your scar becomes the trophy that you survived. The gentle breeze at your back, moving you forward in the direction you want to go. Taking all the time you need.

"Now, as you are ready, coming all the way back, gently tapping, like the beating of a heart, breathing in that **confidence** as you notice that incredible **inner strength**—strength you may never have known you had—the strength that allowed you to go on, despite everything that happened to you and your family."

As Owen's head lifted, and he looked into Mzee's kind, gentle face, there was a big hippo tear on his cheek.

Mzee nodded knowingly and said, "Yes, Owen, what happened to you was very sad. You can't change what is past. Like the river, your life flows forward into the future, leaving what is past behind. I don't know why your whole family was lost, or why you were the only one to survive, but I am so happy that you did, that you were saved, and are here with me now. I feel so lucky to know you, and have you as my friend."

In his imagination, each day, Owen practiced what Mzee had taught him. Days, and then weeks passed, as Owen began to feel stronger and braver. He realized that it was okay for him to smile, to laugh, and have fun. It felt good. Owen was very happy to have found such a wise and wonderful friend. Together they decided to go for a swim.

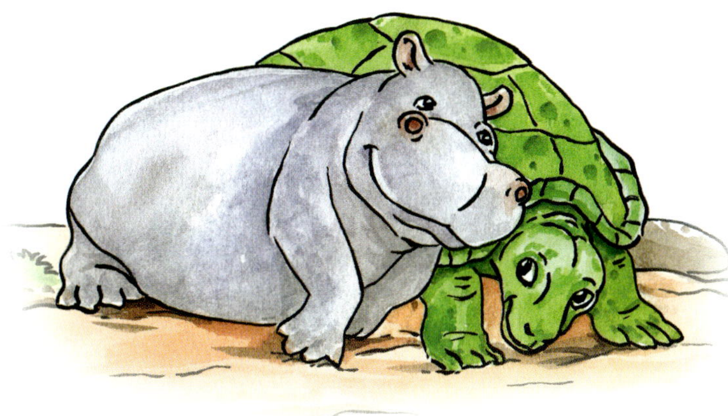

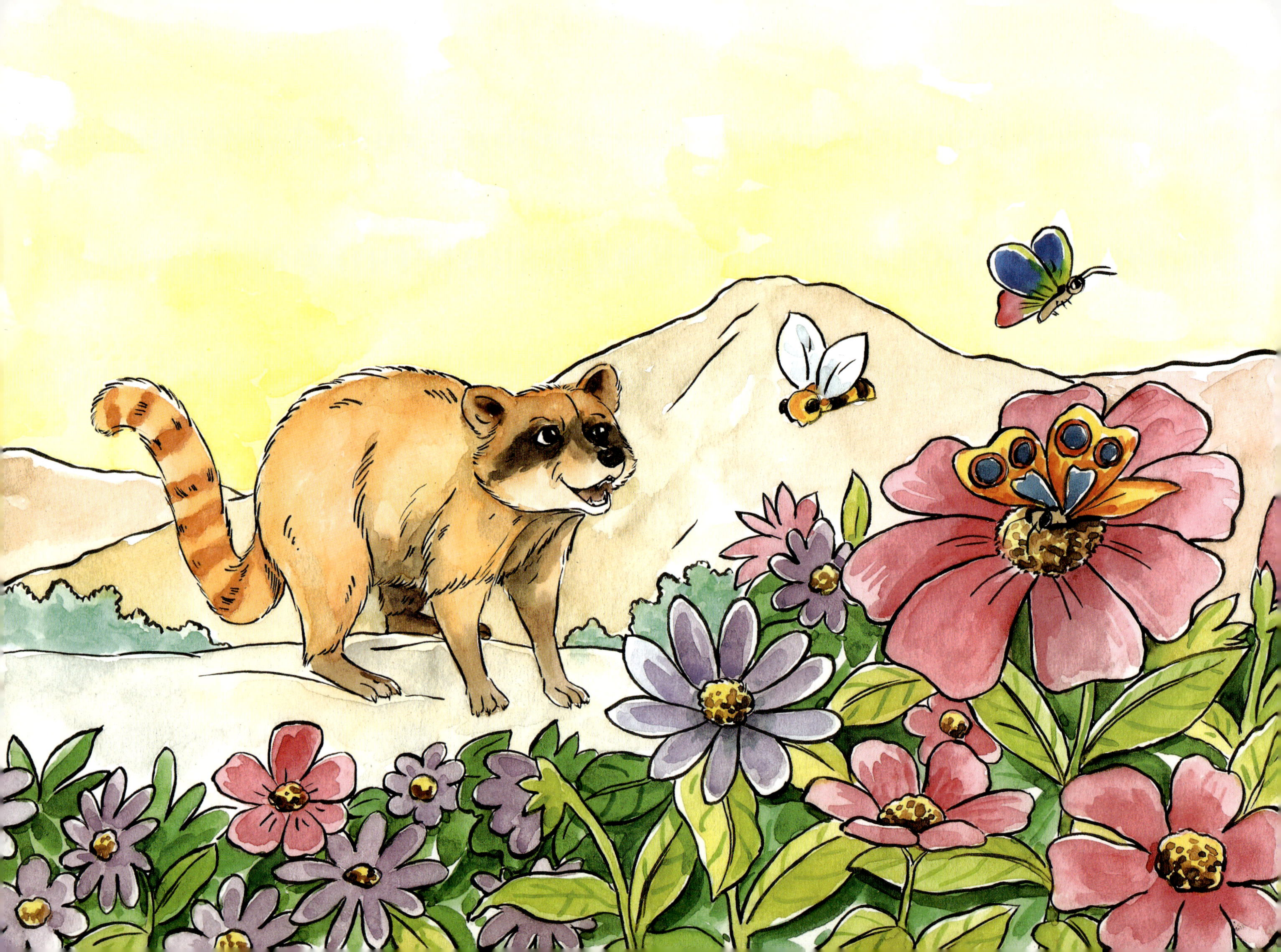

Bloom Raccoon

Bloom was a raccoon. Everybody called him "Bloom" because he loved flowers. The little raccoon didn't care if they were big blooms or small blooms, red blooms or yellow blooms, he loved them all. His favorites were the blossoms that smelled nice.

One day, as Bloom was taking a big sniff of a very big blossom, a bug went right up his nose. Bloom sneezed. Being snuffed up Bloom's nose certainly scared the little bug, and it terrified Bloom. He decided right then and there that he hated bugs. Pretty soon, all flying bugs scared him; then, crawling insects frightened him. Finally, even the beautiful butterflies made him run for cover.

Bloom's fear grew bigger and bigger. Dr. Dan, the Ashland Zoo's veterinarian, called Bloom's big fear a phobia because it got in the way of something Bloom had always liked to do. The little raccoon stopped walking through the zoo's flower gardens. Finally, he stopped going out at all because he was terrified of seeing a bug.

When spring came and all the beautiful flowers in the zoo began to bloom, the little raccoon knew that he needed help.

"I want to be the boss of my fear," he said to himself. "I want to smell the flowers again and not be afraid."

So he went to see Dr. Dan.

Dr. Dan told Bloom, "If you are ready to be the boss of your fear of bugs, then I can help you."

"I certainly am ready," Bloom replied.

Dr. Dan suggested, "You might like to imagine a beautiful garden full of all your favorite flowers and fruits. To keep out all of the bugs, you can create, in your imagination, a huge screened area around your imaginary garden.

"Then, take a moment to really enjoy your garden, the brilliant colors of the flowers: reds, blues, yellows, and pinks. Breathe in the fragrant smells of the flowers one by one … That's right … Now, in your imagination, see and smell the fruits. I wonder which fruit you will decide to enjoy first. Notice how good it tastes.

No bugs, just the beautiful flowers and fruits … Time passes, and now the garden doesn't look so beautiful anymore. There aren't many flowers, and there are very few fruits.

"Don't forget," said Dr. Dan, those beautiful butterflies, bumble bees, and bugs help move the pollen from flower to flower. Without them, there wouldn't be any flowers, and the blossoms on the trees would not turn into fruit.

"You might like to go back to a time before your fear of bugs began.

"Feel again the way you felt when bugs didn't bother you … That's right … Since your imagination makes all things possible, go from 'back' to 'before' to 'forward,' moving forward to the future, … free of your fear of bugs, … feeling proud, … successful and happy. I wonder how interesting it will be to return now in your imagination to the garden with few flowers and not many fruits, and let just one or two butterflies in."

Bloom imagined just two butterflies gracefully and gently fluttering from flower to flower. He noticed, as one lighted on a petal, how truly beautiful the butterfly was. Bloom felt calm and comfortable, so he let in a few more butterflies in his imagination. Then, he decided it would be alright to open the screen to a few bees. The bees paid no attention to Bloom. They were too busy doing bee business, moving pollen from plant to plant. Bloom noticed that the garden was looking better and better. New flowers were beginning to bud, and fruit was ripening on the trees.

Bloom was excited. There were butterflies and bees in the garden of his imagination, and he felt calm and in control, just like he did back before the fear, and just how he wanted to feel in the forward future.

Bloom decided to make the present and the future happen now. He let all the bugs into the garden of his imagination. The blossoms bloomed brighter, and the fruit grew sweeter. The little raccoon was so happy! He was the master gardener of the garden of his imagination. The fruits of his garden were sweet and wonderful. He was the boss; he was in control of the fear he used to have.

Bloom realized that, in an instant, a belief that he used to have—that bugs were scary and bad—could just disappear, and in place of that old belief would be something great. Letting go of fears made room for much better stuff. Bloom's phobia, that old belief that got in the way of what he liked to do, was gone.

Bloom had learned hypnosis—a way of using his imagination to help himself.

Dr. Dan said, “I wonder what other good and useful ways you will find to use hypnosis to help yourself?”

Bloom smiled, but he did not answer. He was too busy sniffing flowers.

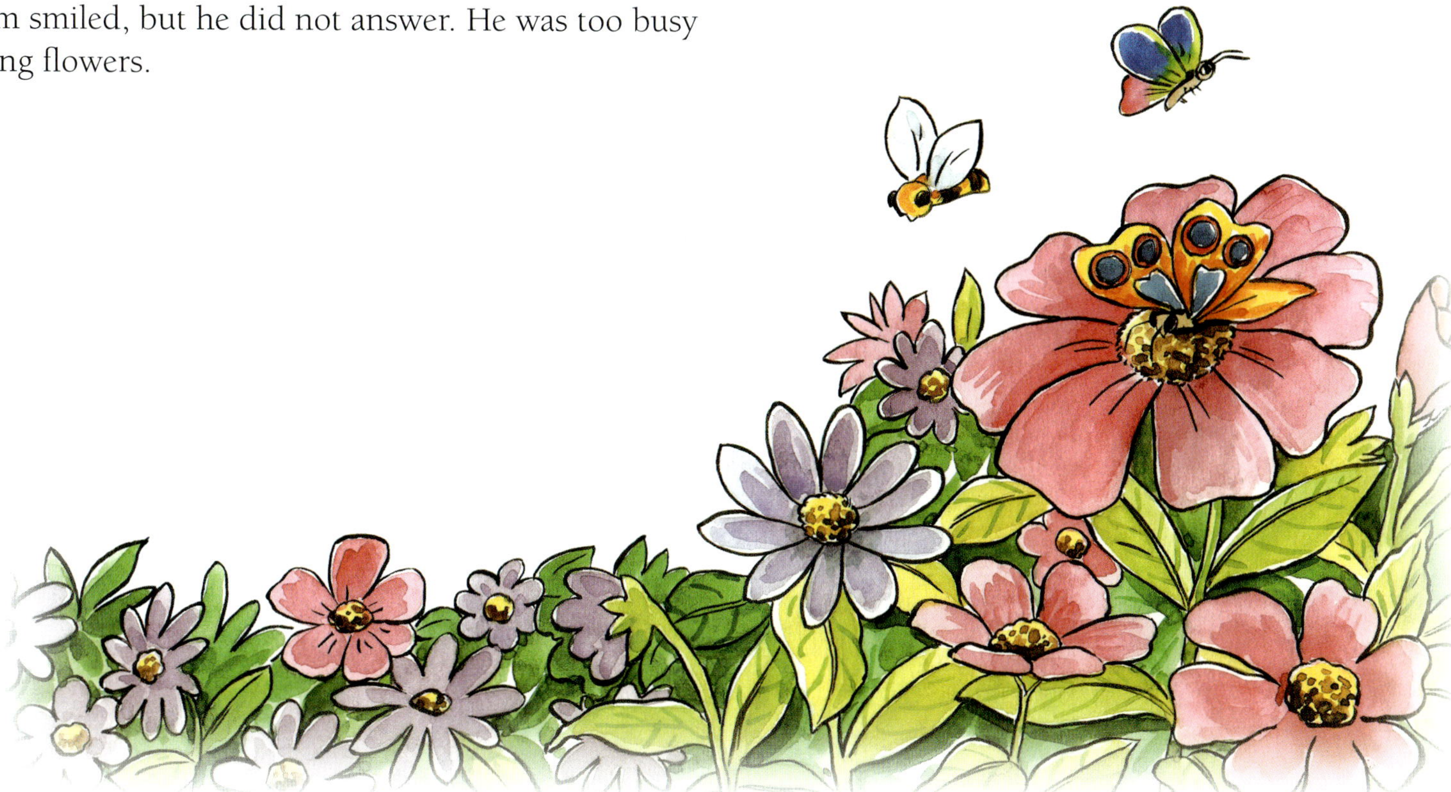

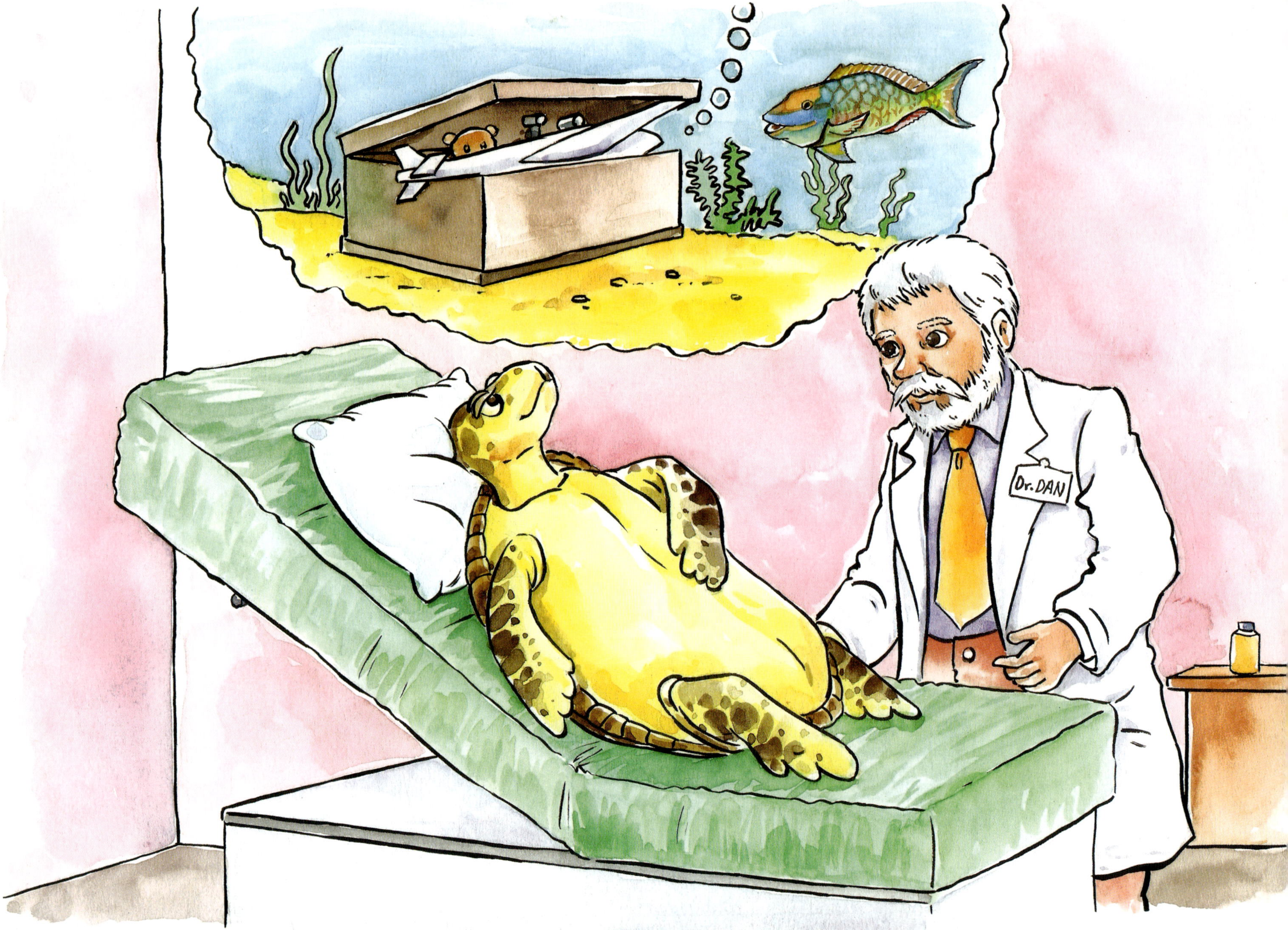
Dr. DAN

Elvira the Green Sea Turtle

Elvira, the green sea turtle came from Costa Rica. She was hatched from a rubbery round egg that her mother laid on a sandy beach next to the Caribbean Sea. The egg that Elvira came from was buried in a very warm place in the sand. Turtles hatched in warm, sandy places are girls. The eggs that hatched Elvira's brothers came from a cooler place in the sand.

As soon as Elvira came out of her eggshell she headed for the sea. She swam hundreds of miles away in the ocean. After twenty-five years, if she was very lucky, Elvira would return to the same beach where she had been hatched to lay her eggs. There are many dangers for young sea turtles. Only one in ten thousand will survive until she is big enough to lay her eggs in the same place where she was born.

Dr. Dan, the Ashland Zoo's veterinarian, met Elvira one starry night while he was on vacation in Tortuguera. *Tortuga* is the Spanish word for turtle. That is how this small town got its name. Dr. Dan watched Elvira crawl up from the ocean onto the sand to lay her eggs. He knew that the sea turtle had important work to do, and that he shouldn't disturb her.

Elvira dug a hole in the sand about two feet deep. There she would deposit from 100 to 150 eggs. The eggs would be white and about the size of a golf ball.

As Elvira began to lay her eggs, she went into a trance. Dr. Dan was surprised to learn that Elvira already knew all about hypnosis. She used her imagination to visualize all the eggs that would become baby turtles. She was thinking so hard about those babies that nothing bothered her. She didn't notice the people around her, and she didn't notice any discomfort that she might feel from pushing out all her eggs. It was almost as if Elvira's body was there, but her mind was somewhere else.

One day, when Dr. Dan came down to the beach, Elvira told him, "I think I might be sick. I have to pee a lot, and it hurts when I pee. Then, even right after I've peed, I feel like I have to go again."

"I'll do some tests," said Dr. Dan.

When the tests came back, Dr. Dan told Elvira, "You have a bladder infection."

"I think I had one of those last year," Elvira answered.

"Well," said Dr. Dan, "because this has happened to you before, you need to have a VCUG."

"What's a VCUG?" Elvira asked.

"It's a special test," replied Dr. Dan. They will put a tiny tube inside you where the pee comes out. After that, they will put a special dye through the tube into your bladder where your pee is stored. Then, with a special camera, they can see what happens to the dye."

Elvira felt a little scared. "I don't think that I will like that test," she said.

Dr. Dan replied, "Do you remember when you were laying your eggs in the sand? Your body was there, but your brain seemed to be someplace else, so nothing disturbed or bothered you. You were so busy using your imagination, that you didn't notice the eggs coming out of your body. You can do the same thing so that the tube going into your body won't need to bother you. I wonder where you would like to go in your imagination?"

"I love the ocean", said Elvira. "I'd like to go there."

When the day for Elvira's VCUG arrived, Elvira left her turtle body on the table in that special room while her imagination dove down deep into the ocean. She swam past schools of colorful fish. Her favorite was called the parrot fish. Elvira thought the parrot fish probably got its name because it had as many bright colors on its body as Molly Macaw, the parrot, had brightly colored feathers.

Elvira swam past coral and sea grasses that moved gently back and forth. She imagined a treasure chest at the bottom of the sea. Slowly, the sea turtle opened the lid, and there inside were some of her very favorite things. She decided to take them out one by one to play with in her imagination while the doctor was busy finishing her VCUG.

The time went by so quickly that Elvira's special test was finished before she even got to everything in the chest. Elvira knew that the treasure chest was always there inside her imagination, and she could return to it whenever she wished.

Meg Dolphin

Meg was an Atlantic bottle-nosed dolphin. She lived with a group of other dolphins called a "pod." These aquatic mammals have excellent vision and hearing, but they cannot smell. They have small ear openings just behind their eyes. They can also hear with their teeth, which act as antennas to receive incoming sound. Perhaps when dolphins look like they are smiling, they are actually allowing their teeth to pick up sound waves so they can pinpoint the exact location of an object. Another amazing thing about dolphins is that when they sleep, only half of their brains sleeps at one time. That meant that Meg could be half awake and half asleep at the same time!

Dolphins communicate with each other by clicks, squeaks, trills, and whistles. The sound is produced by a muscle in the blowhole on top of their head. These sounds can bounce off an object and return to the dolphin like an echo. The echo allows a dolphin to sense the size, distance, and shape of an object. When dolphins are swimming at night, or in murky water, this echolocation is especially important.

One day, Meg's pod was looking for dinner. The dolphins all worked together. Sometimes the pod would push the fish toward shallow water so they were easy to capture. At other times the dolphins would surround the fish, and then take turns swimming into the middle of the group to feed on them.

One day, when the pod was pushing the fish into shallow water, one of the dolphins in Meg's pod got stuck in shallow water. Meg thought it was her fault.

"I must have sent the wrong click to warn the other dolphins," she said to herself.

After that happened, Meg became so worried and nervous about communicating with the other dolphins in her pod that she stopped speaking altogether. Meg spoke with her mom and her sister, but when she was with the pod, she wouldn't say anything. The other dolphins thought this was weird. Sometimes they made fun of Meg. Occasionally, they would play tricks on her just to see if they could get her to speak. This only made Meg more determined not to say anything.

Although she was silent when she was with the pod, Meg was very good at doing the tail walk. She did it so well that she was chosen to be in the Ashland Zoo's dolphin show. The dolphin show was always a favorite with visitors who came to the zoo. Trainers at the dolphin school worked with these aquatic mammals as they breached out of the water, walked backwards on their tails, and sometimes splashed the guests.

The visitors also loved to hear the dolphin sounds, but Meg didn't make any. Although she was silent when she was in the pod, Meg was very good at doing the tail walk. She did it so well that when she came to Ashland Zoo, she was chosen to be in the dolphin show. For her, it had become much easier not to talk than to have to worry about talking. At the dolphin school and show, this was a problem. The dolphins needed to communicate with each other and with their trainer.

The trainer could see that Meg was having trouble. He said to her, "Perhaps Dr. Dan, the zoo's veterinarian, can help."

Dr. Dan was very good at teaching the animals at the zoo how to use their imagination and their own special talents—skills they may never have known they had—to solve their problem by themselves.

"I call it hypnosis," said Dr. Dan. "Hypnosis is learning what you never knew you knew, controlling what you never knew you could."

Dr. Dan asked Meg, "Is being silent a problem for you, one you would like to change?"

Meg shrugged. Not speaking felt comfortable and was easy, while speaking with the other dolphins, and in front of the visitors at the zoo—that was scary.

Dr. Dan said, "You are very good at controlling your voice and not speaking. What other things are you very good at doing?"

Meg didn't want to speak to Dr. Dan, so she just shrugged again.

"I've seen you perform in the dolphin show," said Dr. Dan. "I know how good you are at bursting out of the water and moving backwards while you balance on your tail."

Meg grinned. She was very good at that, and she knew how much the visitors at the zoo enjoyed watching her do it. They always cheered and applauded.

Dr. Dan suggested that Meg take some slow, **deep** breaths through the blowhole on the top of her head. "Find a **comfortable** place. As you breathe in … and

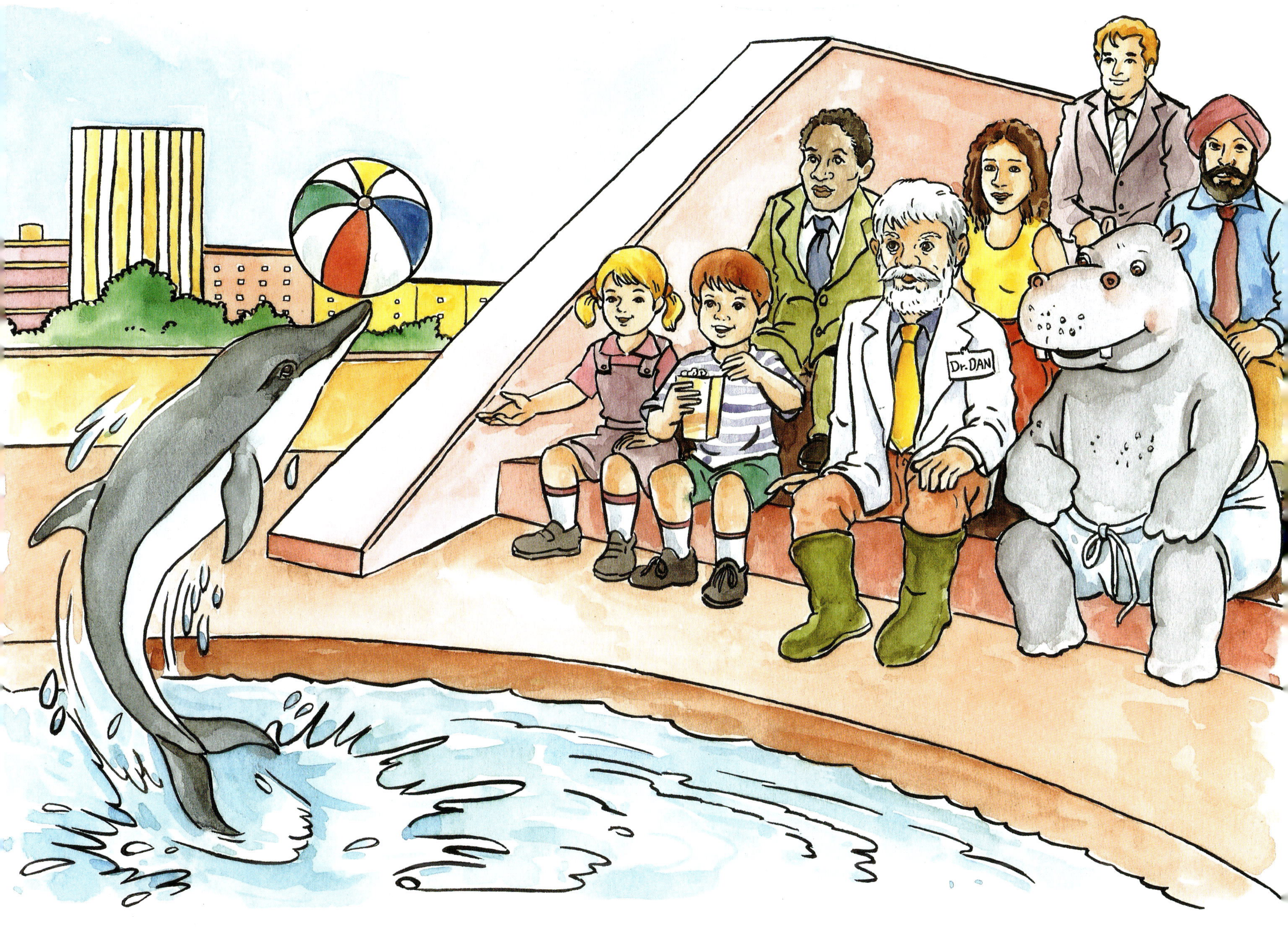
Dr. DAN

as you breathe out—spread the **comfort** through your body … Breathe in **calm** … and as you exhale … let that calm flow through you … That's right … Very **good** … Breathe in **strength** … and allow it to move to all parts of your body as you let go of the breath … Breathe in **confidence** … and feel it grow as it goes from your nose to your toes."

Meg giggled and said, "Dolphins don't have toes." She let out a little gasp as she realized that she had just spoken to Dr. Dan.

"Oopps!" said Dr. Dan. "I misspoke when I said 'toes.' Everybody does that sometimes. Isn't it wonderful, though, that you heard what you needed to hear? That reminds me of a story that Norma Beaver told me about two frogs.

"Two frogs are in a pit, trying in vain to hop out. The frogs at the top are shouting, 'It is hopeless! Give up! You can't make it.'

"One frog lies down and dies. The other frog keeps hopping up and hopping up, and finally makes it out. The frogs at the top ask, 'Why did you keep trying when we told you it was useless?'

"The frog answered, 'I'm deaf. I thought you were cheering me on.' "

Meg smiled her big dolphin grin.

Dr. Dan said, "**You may** wish to remember a happy time in the past when you spoke easily and freely with your friends. **You may** decide to remember how comfortable it is for you to speak with your family. **You may** let your imagination go easily into the future, when speech comes magically, without thinking, almost automatically. Whatever happens, **you will** notice how good it feels to be rid of that old worry. Think about this change, and realize how it will make your life different … better … always … now. Breathe in that **comfort** … breathe in that **calm** … breathe in **confidence** … Good, **very** good."

Meg imagined the crowds at the dolphin show cheering her success as she clicked and spoke her dolphin sounds to the delight of the visitors and all the other dolphins. Mostly, she noticed her own delight—that she could control her worries and anxiety about speaking.

After meeting with Dr. Dan and using her imagination to pretend she was using her voice with others, Meg decided to pretend that she wasn't just pretending. She decided to do it, to go for it. First, she chose a few good friends and spoke with them. She was surprised to discover that it was much easier than she had ever thought it would be. She breathed in confidence, and she felt proud and ready to use her voice in the dolphin show.

Dr. Dan was in the audience as Meg clicked, trilled, and whistled. Dr. Dan's smile almost matched Meg's wide dolphin grin. She had solved the problem she used to have herself, and it felt wonderful.

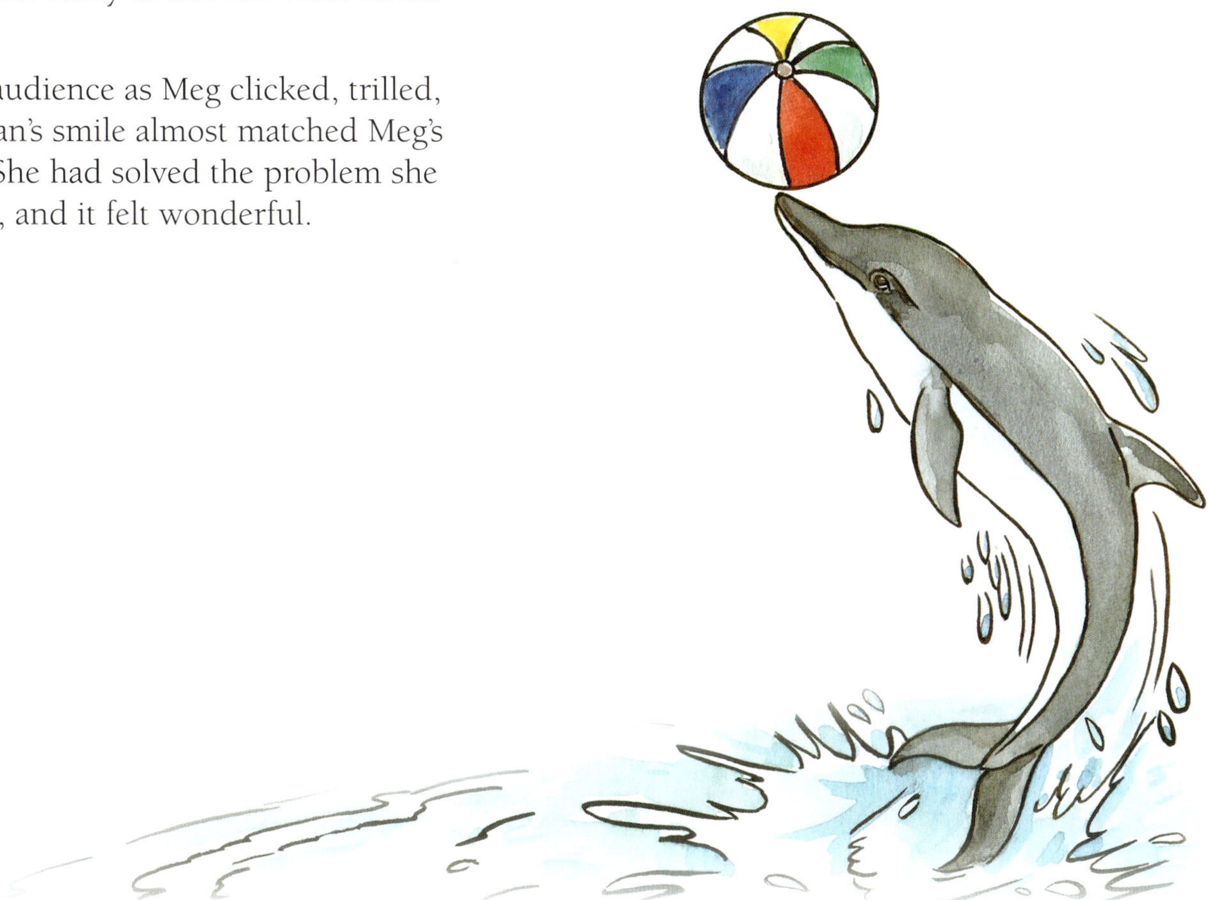

Wester Wallaby

Wester was a yellow-footed rock wallaby. He came from the mountainous rainforests of Australia. Kenzie Kangaroo was Wester's cousin, but you would never guess that because wallabies are so much smaller than other kangaroos—only about the size of a rabbit.

Like his cousin Kenzie, Wester had lived in his mother's pouch for many months. The wallaby's fur was mostly gray, except for on his belly where it was white. He had big yellow feet and a striped yellow tail. Wallabies like to eat grass and live high up on rocky ledges. They are very good at moving quickly over the rocks using only their back feet and powerful tails.

Wester lived in a big colony with about fifty other wallabies. When these little animals sense danger, they bound over the rocks to get away. Young wallabies like to play hide and seek and tag on the high rocks. Wester was afraid of heights, so this was a problem for him. When Wester played high up on the rocks with the other wallabies, he didn't like the way his fear made him feel.

Wester talked about these feelings with his good friend, Harry Hypno-potamus.

"Sometimes it feels like I can't breathe," Wester said. "My heart beats really fast, and I feel sort of shaky."

"I know how you feel," Harry replied. "When the zoo was moving me to a new home, I was scared. My tummy felt yucky. Dr. Dan, the Ashland Zoo's veterinarian, helped me to help myself with brain power exercises that he called 'hypnosis.' "

"Hypnosis? What's that?" the wallaby asked.

Harry answered, "Hypnosis is a way to use your imagination for good stuff instead of worrying about make-believe scary stuff."

Wester went to visit Dr. Dan.

"When I get up high on the rocks, I feel panicky," the wallaby told Dr. Dan. "I want to play hide and seek and tag with the other wallabies, but my fear gets in the way."

Dr. Dan nodded. "So your inside inner fear interferes with fun stuff?"

"Exactly!" Wester replied excitedly. "Could you teach me some brain power exercises so I could help myself with my fear?"

"Get very comfortable," Dr. Dan suggested, "and hold out both your paws. Imagine that in one paw you are holding a very heavy bucket full of sand. A string tied around your other paw is attached to a beautiful helium balloon that is rising higher and higher. I am not sure which paw holds the bucket and which one has the balloon, but you will be able to tell because one will feel very heavy and the other will feel very light. I wonder which sensation you will feel more—the lightness or the heaviness."

Wester closed his eyes so he could experience the balloon and the bucket even better. His right paw began to bend under the weight of the imaginary bucket full of sand.

"Ah," commented Dr. Dan, "I see it is the paw with the heavy bucket of sand that you feel the most.

"Go ahead and pretend that someone is pouring even **more** sand into the bucket, making that paw even **heavier** than it was before. That's right, even more **heavy**. Gently moving **down** to a very **comfortable** position … Now, imagine attaching a second helium balloon to your other paw. Feel twice the lightness. Feel your paw lifting. **Good**. Lighter and lighter."

Wester's paw was slowly rising.

"Now, cut the strings on the balloons, and allow that paw to drift gently and slowly **down** into **comfort**.

"In a moment, if you would like to become even **more comfortable**, even more **relaxed** than you are right now, I am going to ask you to open your eyes. When you close them again, you may be surprised to notice that you are **twice** as **relaxed** as you were the moment before.

"And now, while you are here **safe**, and nicely **relaxed**, imagine watching yourself on a television screen being high up on the rocks and watching the other wallabies play tag. Only experience a little bit of how you feel.

"You may want to talk to me while you are using your hypnosis. Or, I know you remember how to … nod your head 'yes' … Have you forgotten how to shake your head 'no'? … Good.

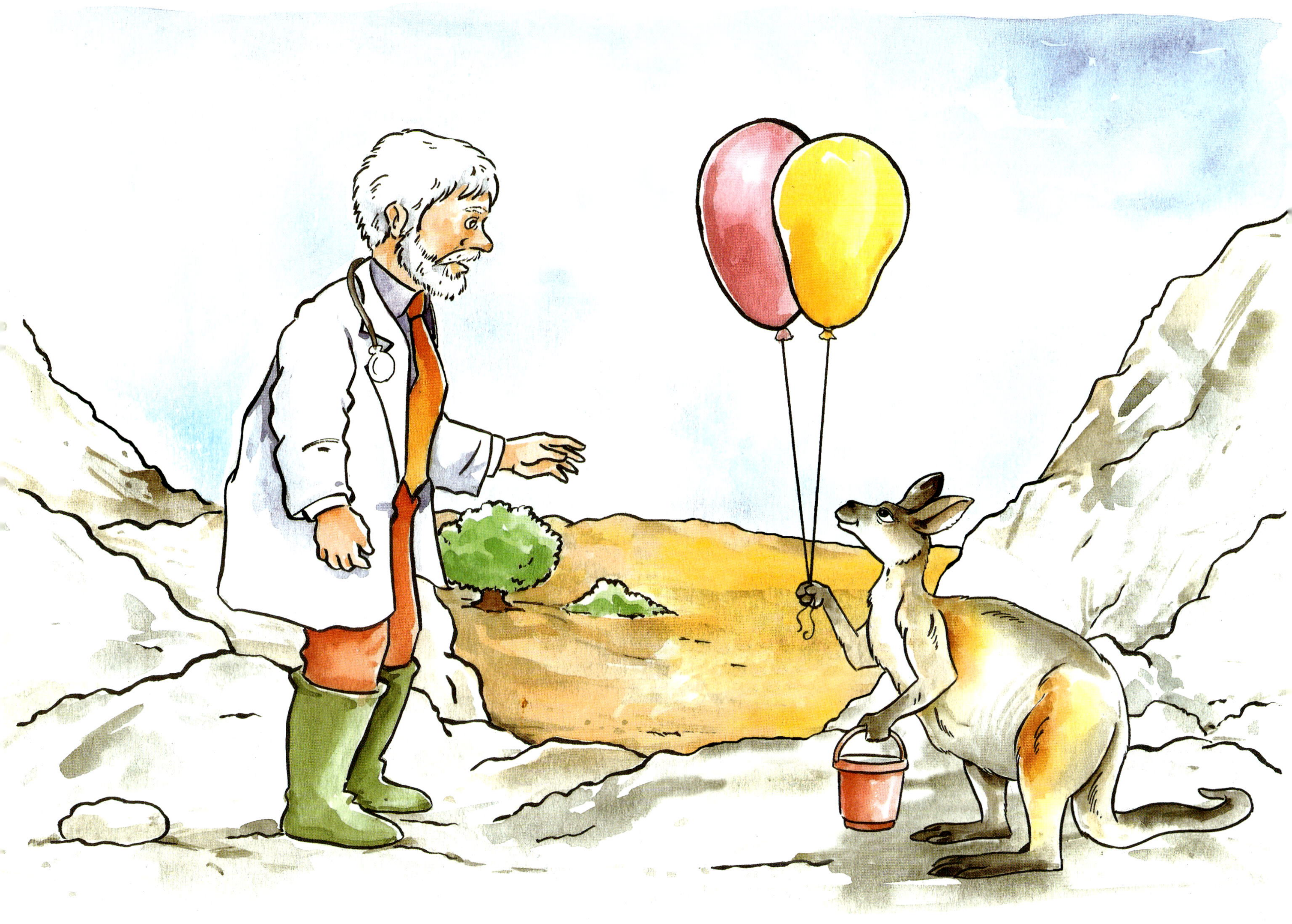

"Now you have choices: to speak with me, or to let your head signal me."

As Wester watched on the screen of his imagination, he began to feel his heart beating faster, and he felt a little like he couldn't breathe.

"I feel nervous and shaky," he told Dr. Dan.

"Breathe in s l o w and **deep**, and then breathe out even slower, breathing **way down deep** into your belly … feeling your belly button rise as you breathe in … and sink **down** into **comfort** as you slowly breathe out … letting your breath **calm** your breathing … That's right. **Very** good. Remembering fear is only a thought. It's not real."

Wester calmed and slowed his breathing.

"Now, feel your heart beating slower as your whole body **calms**. Excellent … **Relaxing** more and **more**."

Dr. Dan noticed Wester's head nodding up and down in agreement.

"When you are ready, but not before you are ready, **now**, watch the screen again as you breathe in new **confidence**. You may wish to blow the fear out into a balloon, and then tie a very tight knot."

"I'm going to pop that balloon," said Wester.

The wallaby began to see the fear he used to have on the screen of his imagination. It looked like a very ugly ogre. Wester decided the ugly ogre fear was not getting the best of him.

"Out ogre, out!" he shouted. "I am stronger than you are. I am the boss of my body and my imagination," the wallaby said with determination.

Wester breathed in strength as he got stronger and more confident, and the ugly ogre got smaller and weaker.

Now Wester was ready to watch himself on the screen of his imagination as he joined the other wallabies playing high on the rocks. Wester began to join in, then stopped and backed up.

"That's okay," said Dr. Dan, "Retreat is okay; it's not a failure … Gather strength … Out, ogre, out. Breathe in … and feel the calm moving through you as you breathe out.

"When you are ready to move forward, and not until you are ready … **now**, pick your foot up from where it has been and move it forward.

"Almost magically, in an instant, the ugly ogre fear you used to have can vanish and be replaced by something wonderful, fun, and lasting."

Wester imagined himself playing with the other wallabies, hopping carefully and easily from rock to rock.

As he realized that he was the boss of his fear, Wester exclaimed, "I love hypnosis! Brain power exercises are great! They gave me the power to conquer the ugly ogre, fear of heights, that I used to have."

Dr. Dan remarked, "I wonder what other new and useful ways you will find to use the brain power exercises that you have learned here today."

"I'll come tell you about them," Wester said, "because now that I know brain power exercises, I'm going to have lots of adventures."

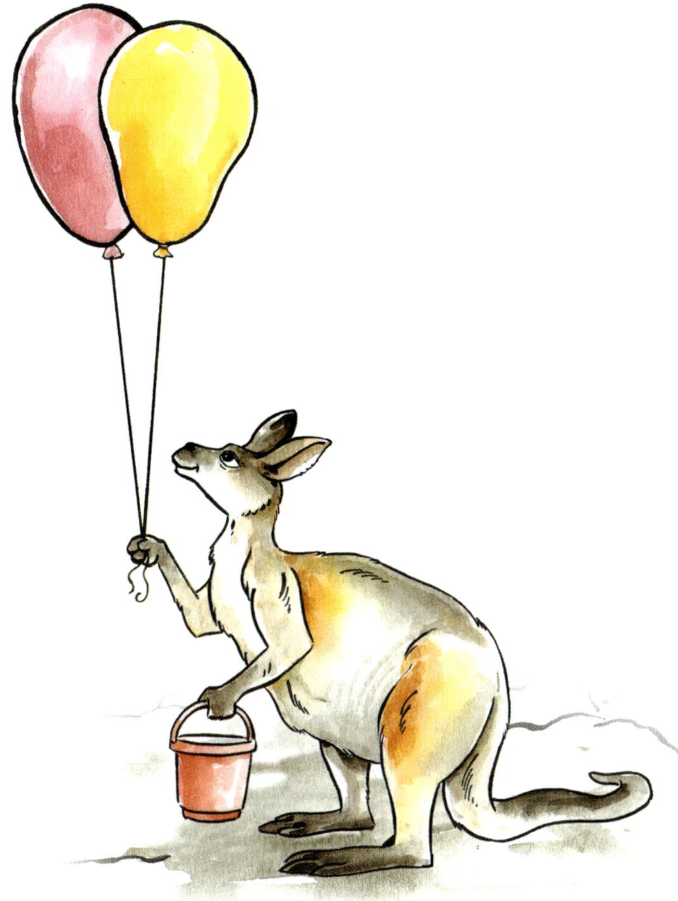

Sam Orangutan

Sam loved trucks. Big trucks, little trucks, dump trucks, fire trucks, tow trucks—he loved them all. Sam was an orangutan. He was four years old, and he still wore diapers. Sam didn't want to go on the toilet. He liked the comforting feel of a diaper on his bottom, so he wasn't sure how it would feel to go on the toilet.

Sam's mother brought him to see Dr. Dan, the Ashland Zoo's veterinarian. Sam didn't really want to discuss what they were there to discuss. He wanted to talk about trucks and play with the toy backhoe that he had brought with him.

Dr. Dan admired Sam's backhoe. "That backhoe is very good at moving things along and depositing them exactly where they need to go," the vet remarked.

"I like fire trucks best, though," said Dr. Dan. Then he told Sam the story of Squirt, the bashful pumper truck.

Once there was a shy pumper fire truck named 'Squirt.' He lived in the fire station with another pumper truck named Flame, a ladder truck named Blaze, and Emily the ambulance. Two police cars also parked inside the fire station. Squirt was friends with everyone who lived there, and everyone liked Squirt a lot. He was funny, and he especially loved making funny faces. Squirt was also kind, he had a great imagination, and he liked helping others.

However, the little pumper truck had a problem: he really wanted to be helpful when there was a fire emergency, but he was too shy and nervous to use his hose to shoot water onto the flames.

All of his friends tried to help and encourage Squirt. Anytime there was a fire, they'd say, "Try to be brave, Squirt!" or "You can do it!" But it never worked. Squirt just couldn't stop himself from being too shy and scared to try. He didn't know how it would feel when the water came out. Would it would hurt, or tickle, or would he feel anything at all? He didn't feel brave enough to find out.

One day, there was a big fire nearby, and all the trucks were called to help. Blaze, Flame, Squirt, and Emily all raced out of the station, with the police cars right behind. At the fire, the trucks all got ready to work, but Squirt was nervous. Blaze, Flame, Emily and the police cars all parked near each other. Squirt felt very sad that he couldn't help.

Blaze looked at Squirt, "It's okay, Squirt. I get scared sometimes, too."

"You do?" Squirt asked. He was surprised to hear someone else felt the same way he did.

"Sure," Blaze said. "Sometimes I'm afraid I won't be strong enough to push my ladder high enough to help. And you know what I do?"

Squirt shook his head.

"I think about all of you who are my best friends at the station, and I imagine that you are all around me in a circle. That makes me feel strong and brave."

Flame moved closer. "You could also use your imagination and see yourself using your hose, putting out the fire, and hearing everyone shout, 'Hooray!'"

One of the police officers got out of their car. "Take deep breaths, Squirt. You will be fine."

"We're all here with you," said Blaze.

Squirt tried, but he still was too shy and too scared.

As all the trucks pulled up closer to Squirt in a circle, Emily asked, "Hey, Squirt, what makes you feel happy?"

"Making funny faces!" answered Squirt. Then he made a face that was so funny his friend, Emily, laughed so hard she snorted.

"Great!" said Emily, who was still laughing. "Now, make faces at the fire!"

Squirt started making funny faces at the fire, and all his friends joined in, making their own funny faces. Soon they were all laughing so hard that Squirt forgot about being shy, and his hose started to fill up with water from his tank. Blaze and Flame made extra funny faces, and the police officers made some of their own. Suddenly, Squirt started to laugh so hard he didn't even realize that water was shooting out of his hose and dowsing the flames!

Flame quickly got his hose going as well, and together they worked to put out the fire!

"You're doing it!" yelled the police officers.

"Hooray, Squirt!" yelled Emily and Blaze. "Keep going! You're doing great!"

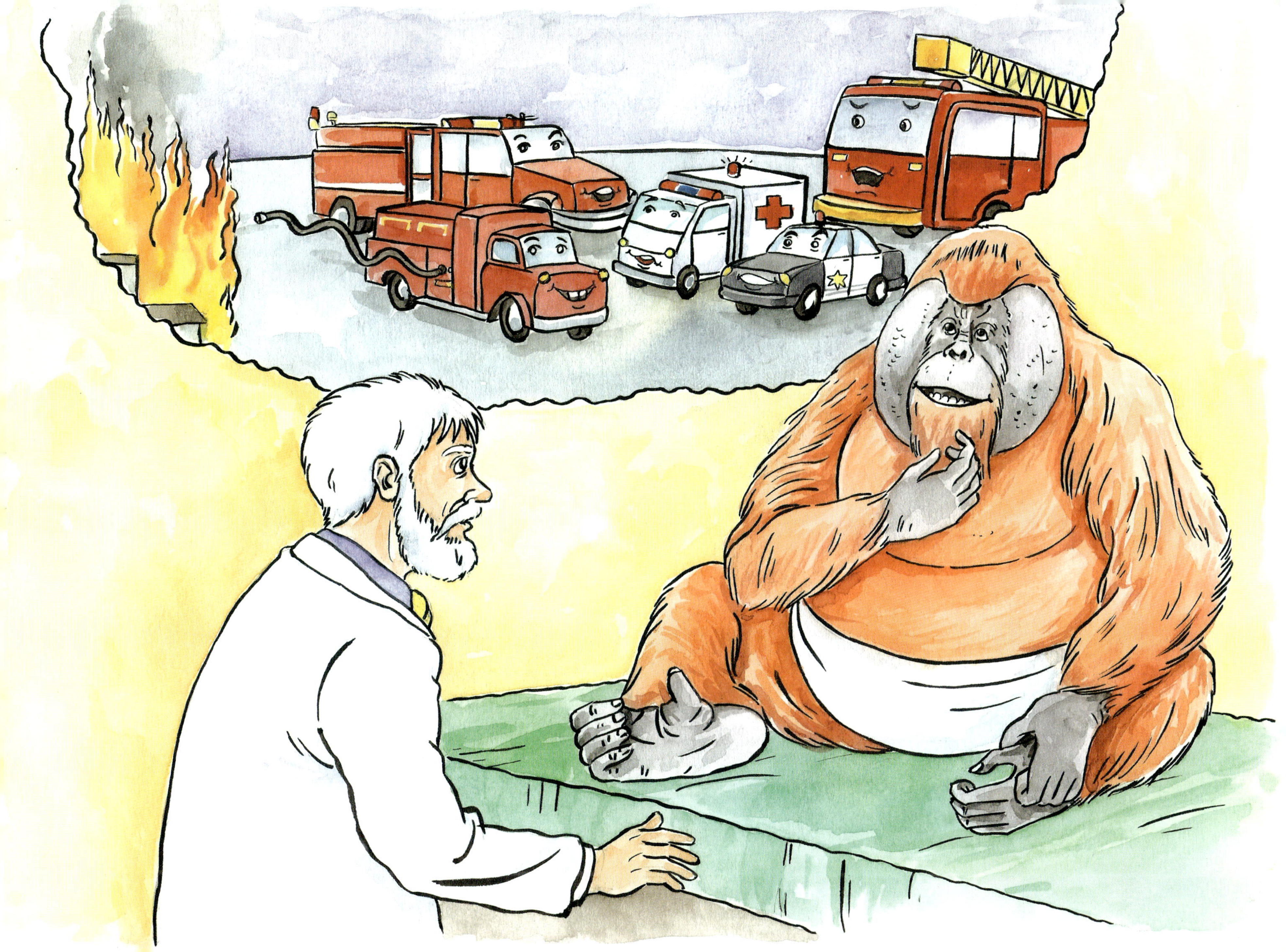

Soon, with Flame and Squirt working together, and all of Squirt's friends parked near him, making him feel brave, the fire was out. Squirt had done it!

"So," said Blaze, "the next time you think you can't do something, or you feel shy or nervous, just imagine all of us around you, making you feel brave, making funny faces, and you'll be just fine."

Flame made one more funny face, and they all started laughing together. Squirt knew he didn't have to feel shy anymore.

Sam thought that he was a lot like Squirt. He was very good at making funny faces, too. He made a great big funny face for Dr. Dan.

Dr. Dan suggested that it might be fun for Sam to pretend that he was the captain of the firehouse. Sam became the boss of all the trucks and their hoses, and soon he didn't need to wear diapers anymore. His funny faces became very happy faces.

Irland Stork

Irland Stork was born in Texas. She had soft white feathers on most of her body except for her tail. Those feathers were greenish black. Irland's long bill and broad, powerful wings made her very good at delivering things. She was so good, in fact, that the Ashland Zoo made her their official letter carrier. She delivered mail and packages to all of the animals at the zoo.

Although Irland was very good at making deliveries to everyone else, the one task that gave her trouble was delivering a pill to her stomach. Swallowing big mouthfuls of fish was easy, but ask her to swallow a pill—no way! It made the stork gag and choke.

When Irland got sick and needed medicine, she had a problem. Some medicines came as liquids that she could sip from a spoon. Others were tablets that could be crushed and mixed with food. Irland was okay with those, but some medicines needed to be swallowed whole, and that is what she thought she couldn't do. The stork was sure that she would choke on the pill before she even tried.

Irland went to talk over her problem with Dr. Dan, the Ashland Zoo's veterinarian.

Dr. Dan reminded Irland, "Ever since you were a baby stork, your body knew just how to swallow, sending nourishment all the way **down** to your stomach, helping you to grow big and strong.

"Imagine now that you have a mouthful of your favorite food. Taste that wonderful flavor in your mouth, rolling your tongue around, tasting every morsel. Notice how moist and slippery your mouth and tongue feels. Now, swallow, as you begin to notice how **comfortably** and **easily** that morsel slides **down** your throat. That's right, **easily** and **comfortably** **down**. I'm not sure what your favorite drink is, but go ahead and pretend that you are taking a great big gulp followed by a **smooth** swallow. Yes, that's right, followed by another gulp and **easy** swallow, going **down** … **effortlessly**. Notice how **comfortable** and **relaxed** all those muscles are in the back of your throat, knowing from the moment you were born just what to do.

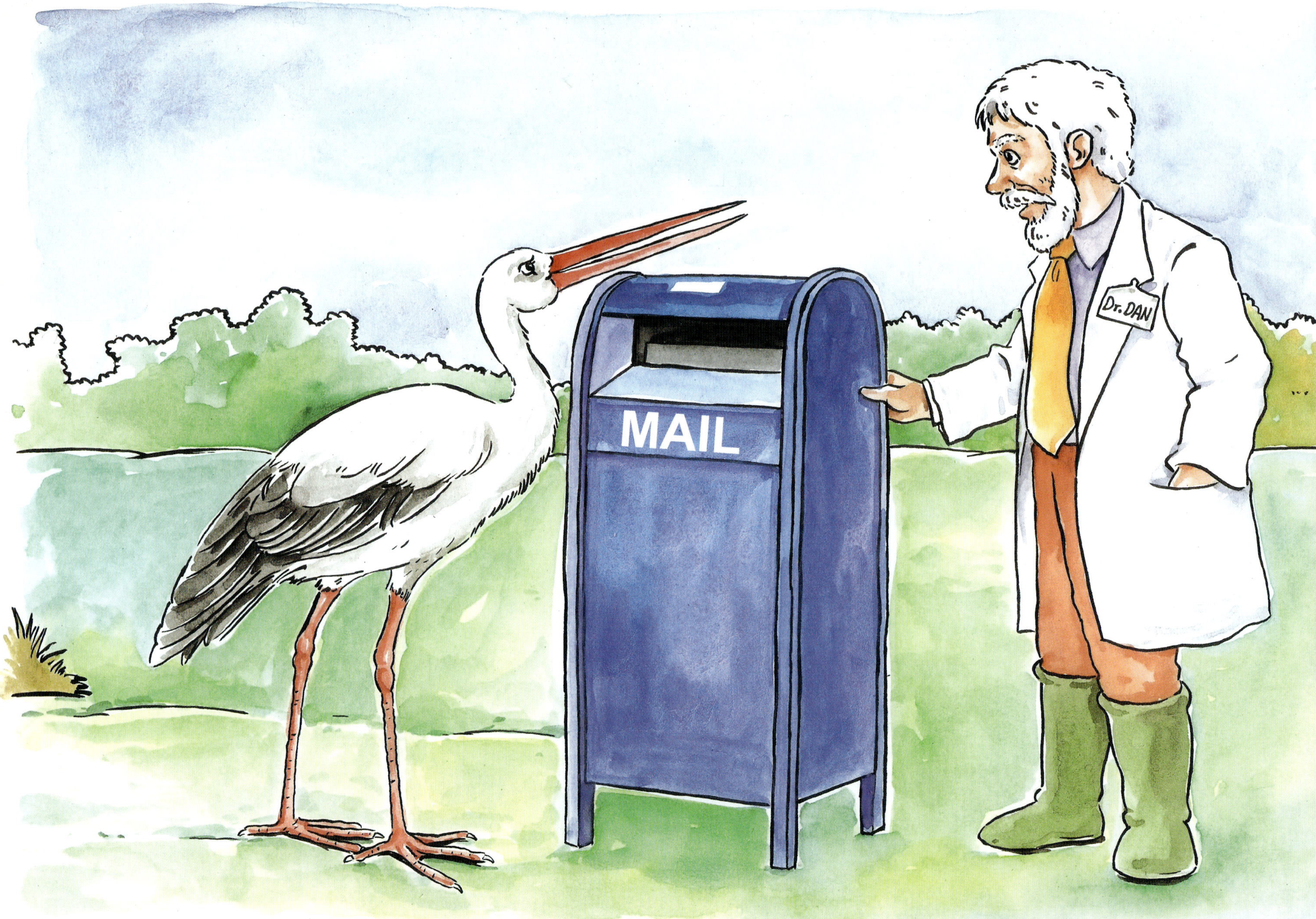
MAIL
Dr. DAN

"Lankton Lizard catches a pill on the tip of his tongue, takes a drink, tilts his head back, and, as fast as he can, swallows. Maggie, the hermit crab, puts her pill in her pincers and tickles her throat as she swallows. Gurgevich Gibbon likes slimy swallows, so he mixes his pills with slippery food like applesauce or yogurt. Sometimes he even pokes it into a banana, takes a bite, then swallows. Oster, the otter, imagines that swallowing a pill is just like a roller coaster. Once the pill gets over the back part of his tongue, it goes down very fast, with gravity pulling it right into his stomach. George Bonobo says that he likes to put the pill in his mouth first and then take a drink. His cousin, Sam Orangutan, says he takes a few swallows of water, holds some in his mouth, pops the pill in, swallows, and—voila!—the pill goes right down. Leora Leopard has a lot of pills that she needs to take. She thinks it is like putting a letter in a mailbox: one swallow, and the medicine disappears, but inside, the pill will be delivered to where it needs to go."

Dr. Dan continued, "In the mirror of your imagination, you can experiment and imagine which way will work best for you, delivering the little pill **gently** and **easily down** into your stomach, and allowing your body to do what it already knows how to do, without thinking, **easily** and automatically."

In the mirror of her imagination, Irland saw herself swallowing pills easily and comfortably. Since she was the letter carrier at the Ashland Zoo and making deliveries was her specialty, she decided to imagine it the same way Leora did. It was like putting a letter into the slot of a mailbox, knowing, as it disappeared, that it would find its way to where it needed to go.

"Now," said Dr. Dan, "we can pretend that you are not pretending. You are doing. I have a mirror, some water, and some M&Ms. The stork stood in front of the mirror and watched as she easily swallowed and rinsed the M&M right down into her tummy. Her long bill curved into a smile.

"I feel so proud!" she exclaimed. "I'm not only good at mail delivery, I can make a perfect pill delivery right into my stomach whenever it needs to be there."

Alter Loon

Alter Loon was born on the shores of Lake Rescue, a small lake in Vermont. Later, it would prove interesting that Alter's parents chose to raise their family on a lake named "Rescue."

Loons eat fish, and they are very good at diving down deep under water to find them. Their big webbed feet are located far back on their body, where they are great for swimming and diving, but not for walking. Since Alter's parents couldn't walk very well on land, they built their nest close to the lakeshore.

While Alter was growing up, he loved his summers on the lake. He loved his peaceful cove. Out in the middle of the lake, noisy motorboats raced across the water. Alter didn't like to wander far from the nest where he grew up.

Summer turned into Fall, and Alter Loon became a grown-up bird. The trees surrounding his northern lake turned brilliant red, orange, and gold, and they began to drop their beautiful leaves into the water. The air felt cool now, and all the children who used to play in the lake were back in school. Lake Rescue was very peaceful, and that made Alter happy. He liked his quiet routines.

One day, Alter's mother said to him, "It's time to leave. You can't stay on Lake Rescue in the winter. You need to fly south, or go to the ocean or a sheltered bay where the water doesn't freeze."

Just like an airplane that needs a long runway to lift skyward, loons need two hundred feet of open water in order to take off and fly.

Alter didn't want to go. His cove felt safe. He liked being there, especially now, with all the motorboats put away for the winter. He wasn't sure what might be lurking out in the world beyond his lake.

The days grew shorter and the nights grew longer. Snow fell, and the lake began to freeze. All of the other loons flew south. Alter was all alone.

Loons have a laughing, yodeling kind of call that they make, especially at night. It is such a eerie sound that people who are thought to be peculiar are sometimes described as "loony," or "crazy as a loon." The families living on Lake Rescue heard Alter's nighttime call and decided that he must certainly be loony.

"What is he still doing here?" they asked each other. "This is Vermont, and it is winter. What will that loon eat once the lake is completely frozen? He won't be able to dive down into the water to catch fish."

Alter began to feel nervous. There wasn't enough open water left on the lake to allow him to take off and fly south.

The men who lived on the lake saw Alter's problem, and they decided to help the young bird. Very carefully, the men went out onto the ice and chopped a hole. They worked at breaking up the ice until there was a two hundred foot runway of open water that would allow the loon to lift off and fly away.

Alter looked at that runway and thought, "It would feel good to stretch my wings."

The loon waddled out over the frozen lake to the runway where he took off and flew. All of the men cheered.

"Mission accomplished!" they shouted.

In a little while it began to get cold and dark. Alter was scared, so he returned to his little cove. By morning, the open water had completely frozen over.

"How can I find any fish for breakfast?" Alter wondered.

The families on Lake Rescue heard his mournful call and said to each other, "We need to rescue that young loon."

When Alter saw his rescuers coming, he was terrified. Then he remembered why his parents had named him Alter. "Alter" means to change.

"Perhaps," thought Alter, "if I can change my thinking, I can change the way I'm feeling and behaving. These people are coming to help me."

The loon grew quiet, so quiet that he could hear what his rescuers were saying.

"We are going to carefully and safely take you to another place where there is open water, other loons, and plenty of fish to eat," they explained.

The rescuers from Lake Rescue gently wrapped Alter in a blanket and drove him to his new winter home.

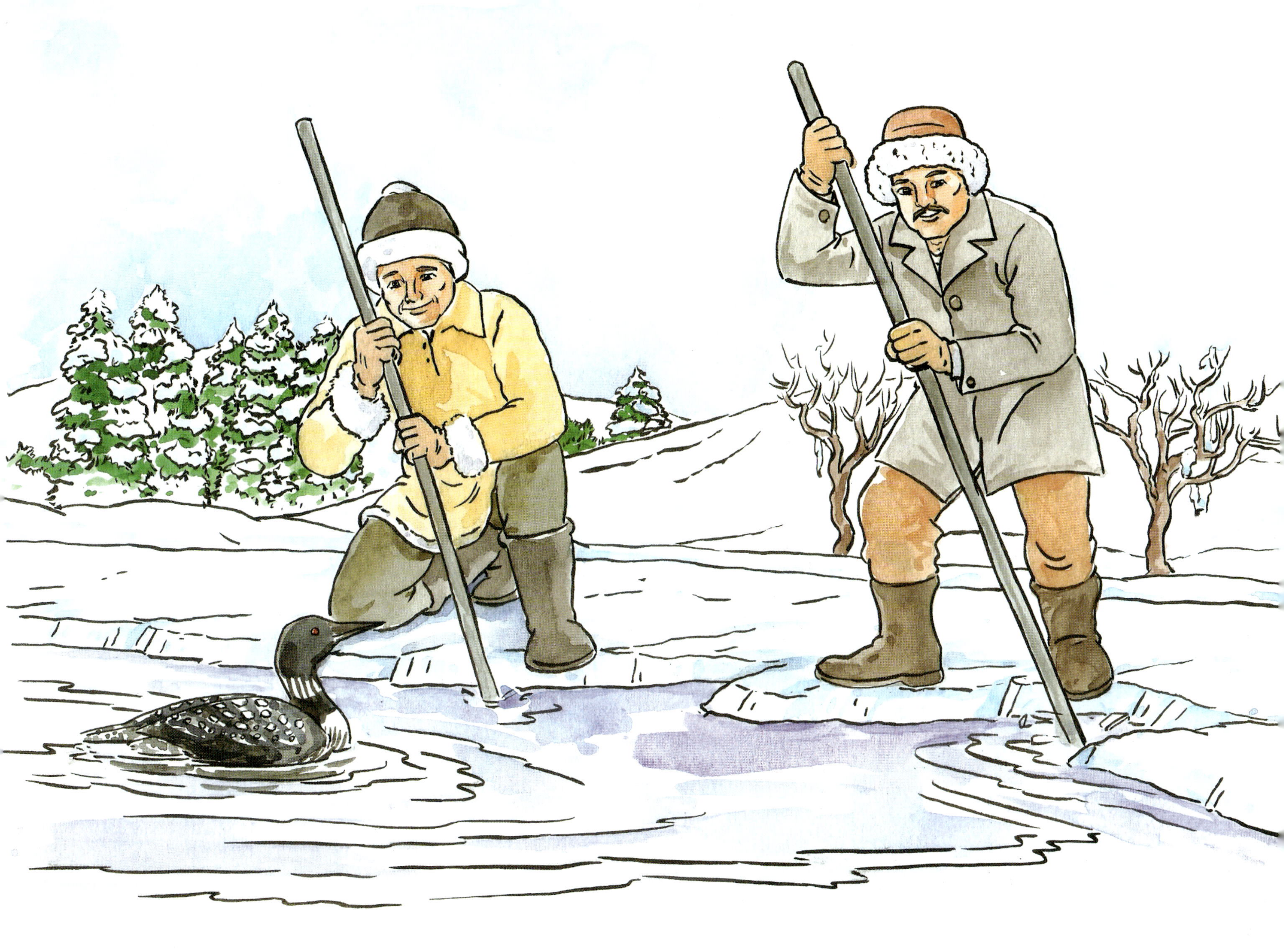

When he got to the new place, Alter felt worried and nervous and scared. He used his imagination to remember his quiet, peaceful little cove, and those memories calmed and relaxed him. Alter began to breathe in new confidence that he had never felt before. He began to "alter" his thinking. This was going to be an adventure! He would see new things and make new friends. Maybe he would even try eating a new kind of fish for supper.

"This isn't so scary after all," he decided. "Mostly, it's exciting. I'll have lots of stories to tell when I go back to my little cove on Lake Rescue next summer."

And the following summer, that is exactly what he did.

Joe Echidna

Joe was a puggle—that's the name for a baby echidna. The puggle came to the Ashland Zoo from New Guinea, a large island near Australia. Like his cousin, Eric Platypus, Joe was a mammal, but he was hatched from an egg the size of a grape. Joe himself wasn't very big. When he was fully grown, he would only be a foot and a half long.

Joe's long, skinny snout, tiny, toothless mouth, and long, sticky tongue were all perfect tools for helping the little puggle get his favorite food—ants. Echidnas are so fond of ants, they are also known as "spiny anteaters." Like a porcupine, Joe's body was covered with prickly spines. He looked pretty scary, but he was actually quite shy.

When Joe was scared, which happened a lot, he could dig a hole to hide in really fast, or he would curl himself up into a spiny ball. Predators wouldn't bother such a prickly ball, so Joe didn't have to worry about that, but there were plenty of other things that scared him. Joe hated storms, loud noises, and the dark, and he worried about lots of stuff. Sometimes his fears and worries got in the way of fun.

One day, the little puggle was telling his troubles to Harry the Hypno-potamus. When he was worried or scared, Harry was very good at using hypnosis to help himself.

"Why don't you talk to Dr. Dan, the zoo's veterinarian," Harry suggested.

Dr. Dan asked Joe about his family, his school, and the things he liked to do.

"What I like best," said Joe, "is eating ants and termites."

Dr. Dan also asked the young puggle about his fears and worries. He listened carefully as Joe told him all about them, then he asked, "Would you like to learn to use your imagination for fun stuff instead of fears?"

"How would I do that?" asked Joe.

"I could teach you about hypnosis," said Dr. Dan. "I can help you to use your imagination to help yourself, to daydream on purpose, to control the fears you never knew you could."

"That sounds wonderful!" Joe replied.

Dr. Dan said, "Get nice and comfortable, and in your imagination, go to a place that makes you feel **safe** and **secure**. Notice everything about that place: the sights … the sounds … so familiar … so **safe** … so **comforting** … Breathe in the smell of that place, and breathe in that **relaxed**, easy feel. Notice that wonderful **calm** feeling as it flows to all parts of your body, making you **more** and more **comfortable** … That's right … Good … You are doing this very well.

"In your imagination, pretend that a curly slide appears, allowing you to slide **down** and around, **deeper** into comfort … Then, climb the steps of the slide again, slowly, and slide again … **down** and around, even deeper into **comfort**, until you are as **deeply** comfortable as you need to be. There is room for only you on the slide. Any worries need to be left somewhere else. Sliding **down** the slide as many times as you want, or need to … until you are as **relaxed** and **calm** as you want to be … Going **down** and around … Let your head nod to signal me when you are very **deeply** relaxed … feeling **safe** and **comfortable**."

Joe's head began to nod.

"Good," said Dr. Dan. "Your brain is like a computer, so when you are ready to learn how to use your imagination, and these very nice, relaxed, **safe** feelings, to re-adjust the computer in your brain, let your head nod to signal me."

Once again the echidna's head nodded.

"Take your mouse, and click on 'Programs.' See what scary or worried programs are running on your computer, and drag them to the trash, or hit 'delete.' … That's right … They don't need to be there. Now, highlight the files you want to run all the time, such as Pride, Self-esteem, Good feelings … You may want to download some of those onto your iPod, remembering you are in charge of downloading only those you want to hear."

In his imagination, Joe adjusted the computer in his brain, and also downloaded to his iPod, the words he needed most to hear all the time.

Dr. Dan told Joe, "Hypnosis is like a present that you give to yourself. The more you do it, the better you get, and the better the gift. Remember to thank the part of yourself that worked hard to control your fears and worries, and especially thank the computer programmer who learned to control, all by himself, what he never knew he could."

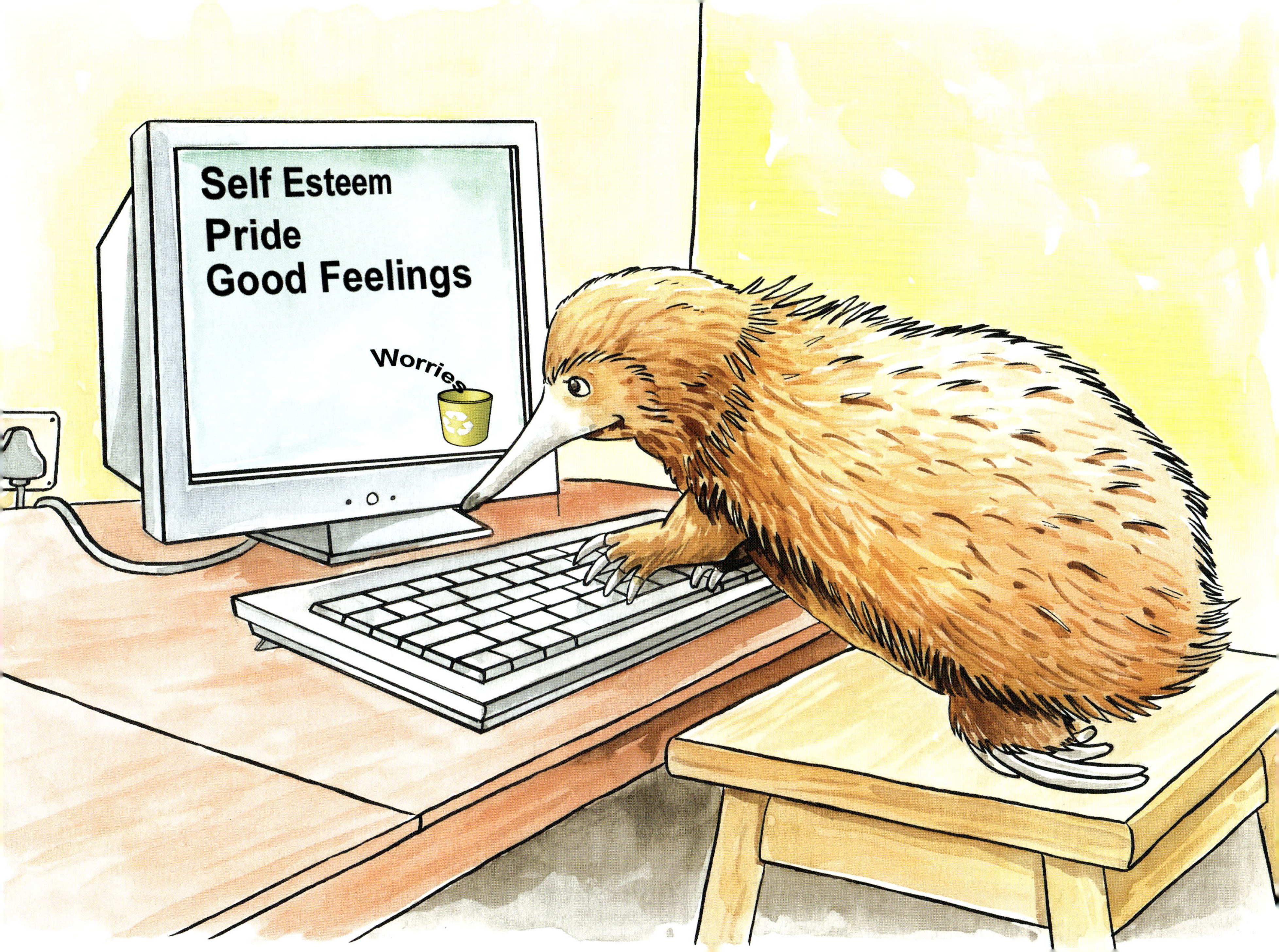
Self Esteem
Pride
Good Feelings
Worries

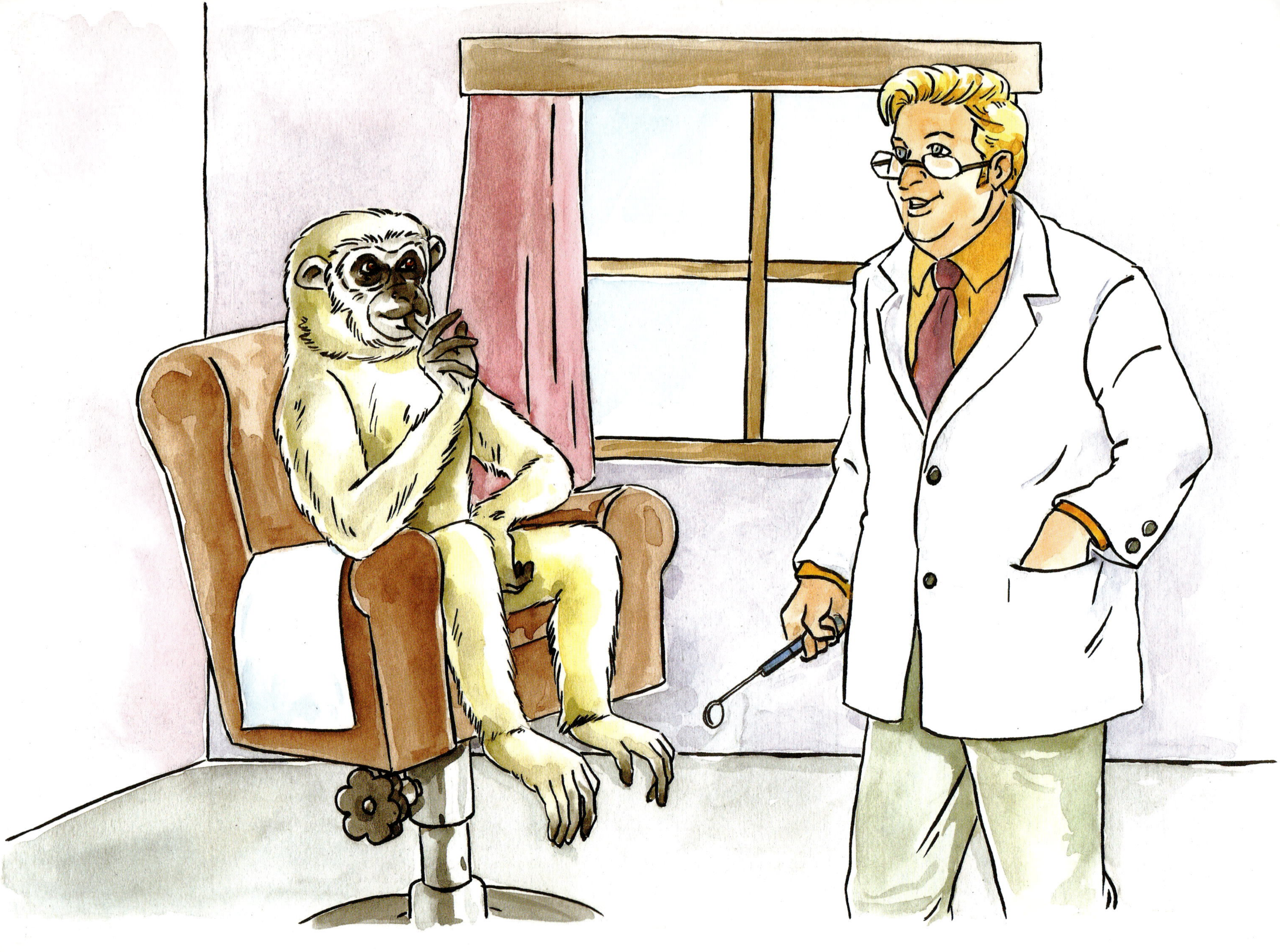

Gurgevich Gibbon

Gurgevich was a gibbon. Before he came to the Ashland Zoo, he lived in a forest in China. Gibbons are the smallest members of the ape family, about the size of a monkey. The little gibbon had very long arms and legs. Harry Hypno-potamus thought the name "Gurgevich" was pretty long, too, so he called him "Gurg." Like all gibbons, Gurg no tail. He used his long arms to swing from branch to branch. That was a problem for the gibbon, because he always sucked one of his fingers. It is hard to swing in the treetops using only one hand.

Dr. Goodman was the Ashland Zoo's dentist. One day, when he was examining Gurg's teeth, he noticed that some of his teeth didn't close just right because his finger was always in his mouth.

He said to Gurg, "I wonder if you like the taste of that one best, because I haven't seen you suck any of your other fingers."

Gurg nodded. "That's my favorite finger."

"Hmmm," said Dr. Goodman, "I wonder if your other fingers would taste just as good."

"I don't know," Gurg admitted, "because I only like to suck that one."

"Would you like to stop sucking your finger?" Dr. Goodman asked.

Gurg said, "It sure would be easier to climb trees and swing from the vines if I didn't have my finger in my mouth. I need all of my fingers to hold onto things. I want to stop, but I don't know how."

Gurg was good at sucking his finger. He could do it without even thinking about it. It had become a habit, something he did over and over so many times that after a while he didn't even realize that he was doing it.

Dr. Goodman asked Gurg, "How would you like to help me with an experiment?"

"What kind of experiment?" asked the gibbon.

"A taste test," answered Dr. Goodman. "Since you have ten fingers, and you have spent your whole life so far sucking on just one finger, it's time to give your other fingers a turn to see what they taste like."

Together the dentist and the gibbon made a chart. Each finger was assigned a different day on the chart.

"During the first week, on Monday," Dr. Goodman suggested, "you can suck the thumb on your left hand as much as you want to, but only that thumb. On Tuesday, you can suck your pointer finger all day. Wednesday will be for your left middle finger, and on Thursday you can suck your fourth finger just as much as you please. Then, on Friday, just before switching to your other hand, you could suck your left little finger all day to see how it tastes. On the sixth day, you would start with the thumb on your right hand, remembering to suck your right thumb all that day. You would finish out the ten days sucking a different finger each day. After that, you could either begin again, or you could decide right away which finger flavor you like the best."

"That sounds like fun," Gurg said.

On Monday, Gurg was about to put his favorite finger in his mouth when he remembered that it was left thumb day. The thumb tasted about the same as his favorite finger, but it didn't feel quite right in his mouth. Several times that day, Gurg's favorite finger began to move toward his mouth. Suddenly, he would remember that it was Monday, left thumb day, and he would stop and suck his left thumb.

Each day, Gurg sucked only the finger that was on the chart for that day. Friday was pinkie day, the day for his little finger. So far, the gibbon didn't think any of his fingers tasted any different. His favorite finger wasn't beginning to move toward his mouth as often. By the following Monday, the gibbon was beginning to forget to remember, or maybe he was just remembering to forget, that habit he used to have. He realized that he was able to control what he never knew he could. He no longer needed or wanted to suck his favorite finger. Gurg was excited about telling Dr. Goodman.

"How did the taste test turn out?" Dr. Goodman asked Gurg.

Gurg laughed and said, "I didn't like the taste of any of them. I'm done with sucking my fingers."

"That's wonderful!" said Dr. Goodman. "I'll bet I know something that would taste good—a banana ice cream cone."

"It sure would," Gurg agreed.

Dr Goodman and Gurg headed off to celebrate. Gurg had stopped sucking his finger all by himself, and that felt great.

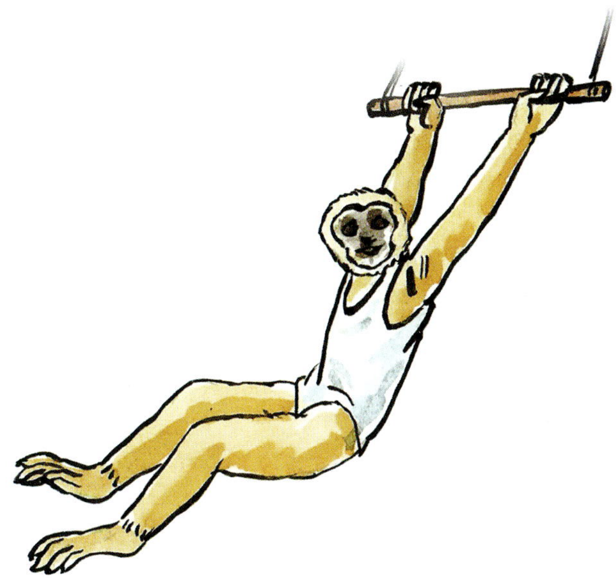

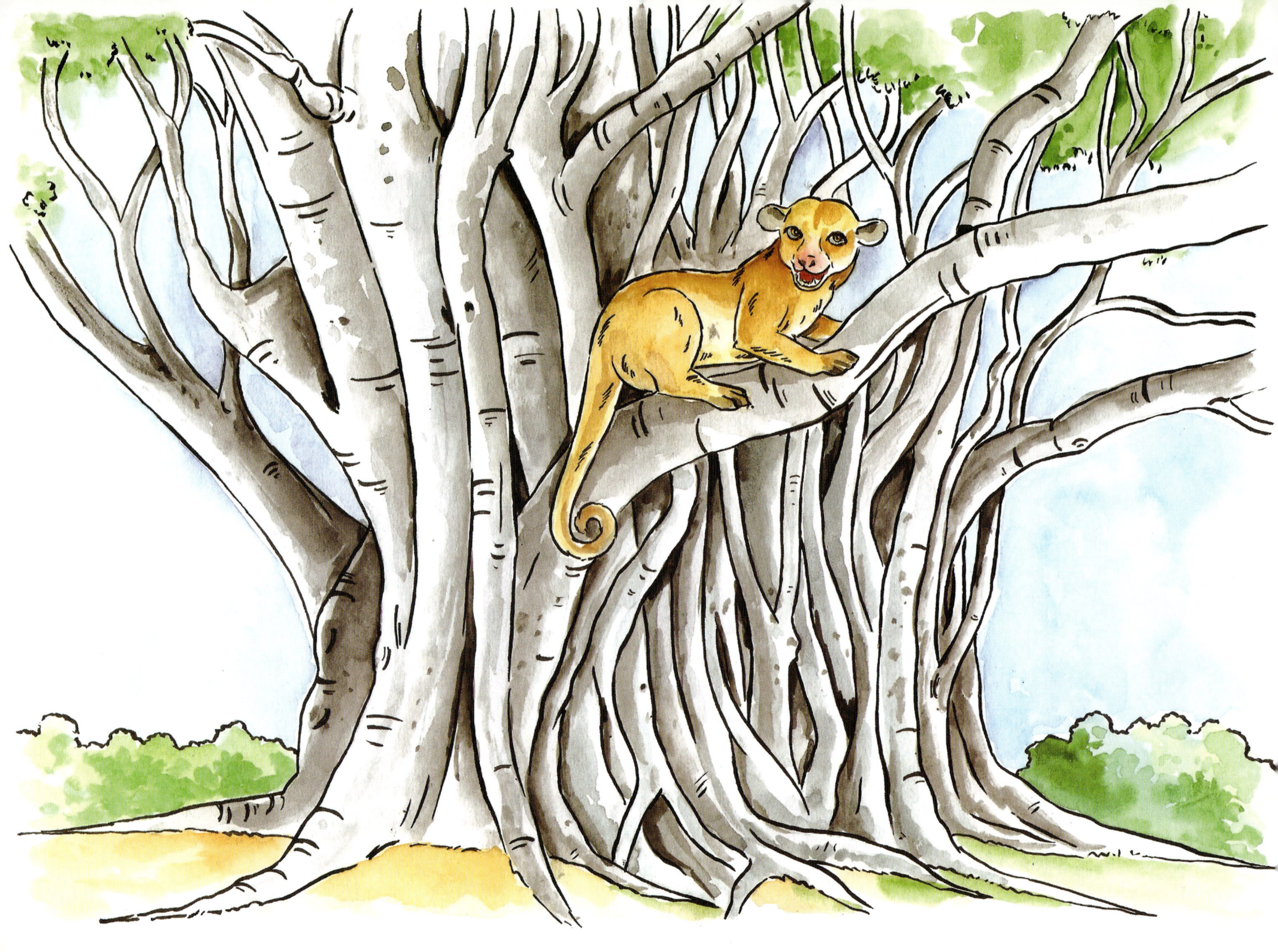

Carol Kinkajou

Carol was a kinkajou. She came to the Ashland Zoo from a tropical forest in South America. Some people call kinkajous "honey bears" because they are round and brown like little bears. Actually, they are cousins to raccoons. Carol was smaller than a raccoon, though. She was about the size of a cat, and she had a long, clever tail that helped her to get around in the treetops of the rainforest. The kinkajou had paws that looked like little hands. At the ends of those hand-like paws were long claws that helped Carol to climb high into the trees. There she found sweet fruits to eat. Not much sunlight gets through the thick trees of the rainforest, but Carol's very large eyes helped her to see in the dark.

One of a kinkajou's favorite things to do is to drink the nectar of the white balsa flowers that grow way up high in the forest. Carol would stick her whole nose and mouth down into the flower blossom and drink the sweet nectar with her long tongue. When she pulled her nose out of the flower, her whole face would be covered with white pollen. Carol moved the pollen from flower to flower as she drank.

One day, as the kinkajou was drinking the nectar of the balsa flower, she took in a big breath of pollen. The pollen tickled the back of Carol's throat, and she began to cough to clear away the pollen.

Even after the pollen was gone, Carol kept coughing off and on. She became very good at coughing and clearing her throat. Soon, the kinkajou was coughing a lot without ever meaning to. This annoyed the other kinkajous. Coughing had become a habit, something that Carol did really well without even thinking about it. She wanted to stop, but she didn't know how.

Harry the Hypno-potamus told Carol, "If you want to control your coughing and throat clearing, Dr. Dan could teach you how to use hypnosis to help yourself."

When Carol went to Dr. Dan's office, Dr. Dan examined her very carefully. He talked with her about becoming the boss of her cough.

"You are not coughing and clearing your throat because you are sick," he reassured her, "and there is nothing wrong with your throat or your chest. Your cough and throat-clearing began for a reason, and then they just got stuck. The reason is no longer important. It has just become a habit."

Dr. Dan taught Carol how to do belly breathing. The kinkajou took a deep breath in through her nose and exhaled slowly through her mouth. She put a hand on her belly to feel it rise and fall with every breath. She began to notice how, each time she breathed out, her throat felt more and more relaxed. Carol breathed slowly and deeply. When she let go of her breath, she also let go of the tightness in her throat. The kinkajou liked belly breathing. It made her feel good all over.

Dr. Dan suggested, "You could go someplace wonderful in your imagination."

Carol remembered her home in the rainforest. In her daydream, she heard the sounds of the rain … so familiar … so safe … so comfortable … and she saw all her friends who lived there. Gently, Carol breathed in the smell of the place and allowed it to fill her with peacefulness.

While she was nicely relaxed and comfortable, Dr. Dan suggested, "You are the boss of your body, just like you are the boss of your imagination. Using your imagination, you can learn to control what you never knew you could."

Habits can sometimes get in the way of fun stuff. Carol wanted to stop her annoying cough and throat clearing. She imagined one of her favorite trees in the rainforest. It was called a golden fig, and the kinkajou loved to eat its fruit. Her animal droppings contained the tiny, sticky fig seeds. The droppings fell on the branches and notches of a host tree, and the seeds began to grow there. Long roots grew down toward the ground. Gathering nourishment from the earth, the new fig tree began to grow strong and tall, wrapping itself around the host tree.

Carol imagined that she was like the small fig tree, and her cough was the host tree that she wrapped herself around. With each breath, the little fig tree gained strength from its roots. The host tree in the middle, that had once served a purpose, began to get weaker and weaker as the fig tree quietly grew bigger and stronger.

Silently, the golden fig tree grew, its confidence increasing as it reached toward wonderful heights. Once, the fig tree had needed that old inside tree, but now, as time has passed, the old habit of growing around the tree was no longer useful. The fig tree had reached its goal: to stand tall, all on its own. The inside tree, no longer needed, began to shrink and quietly disappear. Nothing was left of the tree that used to be. Instead, the fig tree created a wonderful empty, open place that is loved and very important to all the creatures of the rainforest. The golden fig tree is free to be free to reach for the silent stars.

When Carol returned from her very pleasant daydream, she quietly noticed how calm and comfortable her throat felt. Her cough, no longer needed, had silently disappeared.

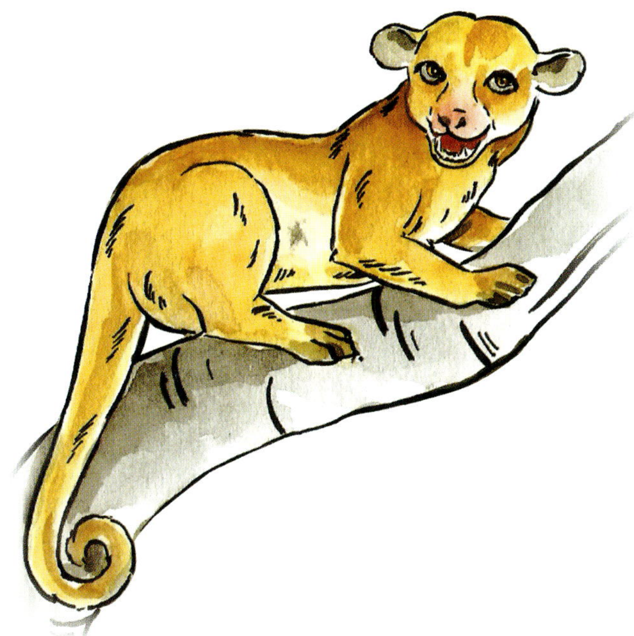

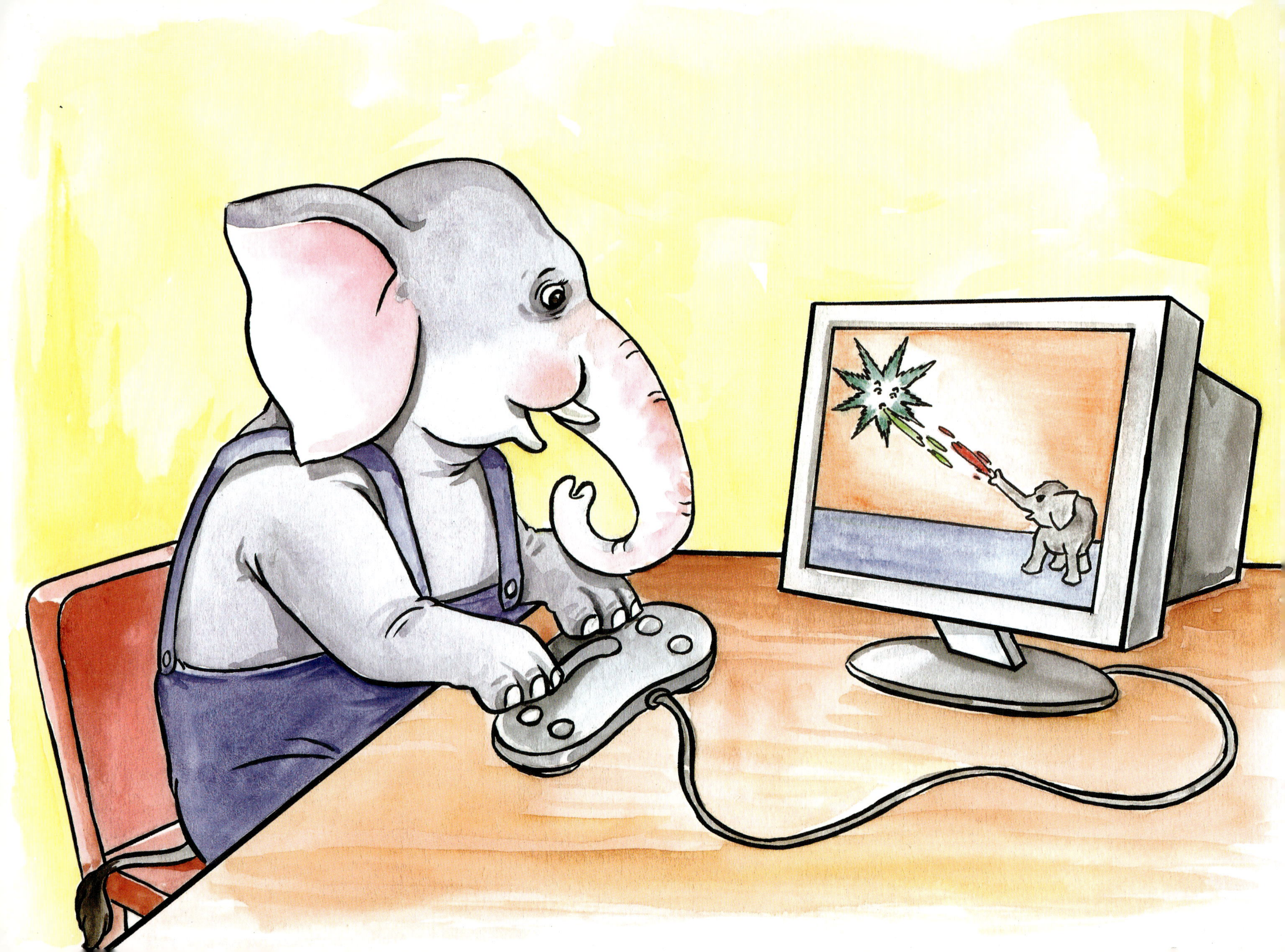

Yapko Elephant

Yapko was an Asian elephant. He looked a little different from Elkins, his cousin from Africa. Elkins had big ears that were shaped like a map of Africa. Yapko was a little smaller than his African cousin. He had small ears and very dry, wrinkled skin.

Yapko had a problem. A very itchy red rash covered most of his body. Since his body was very big, he had a very big problem. The more Yapko's rash itched, the more the elephant scratched, and the more he scratched, the more it itched. Yapko would try to scratch behind his ears with his long trunk. To scratch his side, he would go to a fence and rub his body back and forth. When the top of his head needed a scratch, Yapko would rub it against a tree. Almost anything in the elephant enclosure became a scratching post for Yapko. His skin got very red and sore from all that scratching.

Harry the Hypno-potamus was Yapko's friend.

"I think hypnosis could help," said Harry. "Dr. Dan, the Ashland Zoo's veterinarian, could show you how to use hypnosis to help yourself with your itching."

Dr. Dan came to visit Yapko. "What does the rash feel like when it is bothering you," he asked the elephant, "and what things do you already know how to do to make your rash feel better?"

Yapko said, "The rash is prickly, and it burns. Cool water always makes it feel better."

Dr. Dan asked Yapko, "What things do you especially like to do?"

The elephant said, "Even though my legs are as big as trees, my trunk is very clever. It can pick up something as small as a peanut. I like to use my long, clever trunk to play video games. That's my favorite thing to do."

"Since you are so good at playing video games, I'll bet you could imagine that you are playing your favorite game right now," said Dr. Dan.

"Yes, I can," replied Yapko "and I am already winning!"

"That's wonderful," said Dr. Dan. "Perhaps you are already beginning to notice … or perhaps, in just a moment … **now** … that the itch you used to have is bothering you less and less."

Yapko nodded in agreement as he continued to play the video game in his imagination.

"I wonder how wonderful it would be to design and create your very own video game in your imagination. As you play the game, each win gives you a shower of cool comfort," said Dr. Dan.

"Yes!" Yapko replied excitedly. "It's a purple shower because purple is a comfy color. The shower feels soothing and gentle. It is a contest between me and Itch Man to see who can get to the purple Itchy Switchy first. But if Itch Man pops up, then I can blast him with my red hose and shout, '*Itch Man, no itchy itches*!'"

Then Yapko shouted excitedly, "I won! I got to the Itchy Switchy first and turned it off!"

Yapko was having so much fun creating and playing the new video game in his imagination, he forgot all about scratching.

Dr. Dan said, "Every great video game needs a name. What are you going to call yours?"

"That's easy," replied the elephant, "It's 'YAPKO's KOOL and KOMFY GAME."

George Bonobo

George Bonobo came to the Ashland Zoo from Africa. Bonobos are human beings' closest cousins. They look like chimpanzees, but they are a little smaller and much smarter. George was certainly smarter than a chimp, but he wasn't smaller. For a bonobo, he was very tall.

One day, some visitors to the zoo called George a chimp, and that made the bonobo upset. He didn't want people to think he was a chimp; he was a bonobo. He started to tell them so, but the words came out: "I'm a bbbbbonnnnoBO." That had never happened to George before. He tried again: "BbbbbonnnnoBO." This was embarrassing. George couldn't get the words out without stuttering.

George was the Master of Ceremonies for the animal show at the Ashland Zoo. He worried that he would begin to stutter in front of all the visitors who came to see the show. The more he worried about his stuttering, the worse it got.

George said to Harry the Hypno-potamus, "I dddddddon't know what I am ggggoing to dddddo."

Harry said, "I bet Dr. Dan can help. He is the Ashland Zoo's veterinarian. He can teach you how to do self-hypnosis. That's a way of controlling what you never knew you could."

George went to visit Dr. Dan.

The veterinarian said to George, "Stretch out and get **comfortable**. Imagine that your belly button is a yo-yo, and I've got the string. Your belly button is a very clever yo-yo, and it can do tricks, so watch very carefully. To make the yo-yo go up with my hand, breathe in deeply so it pushes your yo-yo belly button up … Then, as my hand comes **down**, and the yo-yo goes **down**, let your breath out … That's right … Breathe way **down** into your belly as my hand rises, … and then, as my hand moves **down**ward, … exhale very slowly."

Dr. Dan raised his hand even higher, and then down very slowly. "Good. You have a great yo-yo belly button. Perhaps you are noticing that each time the yo-yo goes **down**, you go **deeper relaxed**, becoming more and more **relaxed** … more and more **comfortable** … This yo-yo is so clever, it can even go without the string. So go ahead and cut the imaginary string, and notice how it can go all by itself … slowly … **comfortably**, with your breath."

George liked yo-yo breathing. It made him feel very relaxed and comfortable.

"Now, while you are feeling nice and **comfy**, go to a happy place in your imagination."

George imagined that he was by a little stream in the woods. He noticed how easily the water was flowing in the stream, flowing smoothly around the bends and over the rocks.

Dr. Dan suggested, "From your place of **calm** and **comfort**, imagine that you have a pair of binoculars. As you put the binoculars up to your eyes, you can see all the way to the animal show at the zoo. Binoculars are very interesting. If you hold them one way, things that are far away seem to be up close, and you can see them clearly. When you turn them around and look through the other end, everything looks tiny and far away."

Dr. Dan asked the bonobo to look through the binoculars into the past, before the stuttering, and see and hear himself as the MC of the animal show speaking easily.

"The words flowing smoothly from your mouth, then, still looking through the end of the binoculars that bring things up close and clearly, see and hear into the future, the future free of stuttering … watching and listening as you control the flow of the animal show … master of ceremonies, master of your body and your voice … Yes, that's right … see and hear it happening."

"Now," said Dr. Dan, "look at the present through the other end of the binoculars, the end where things look small and far away. It is difficult to see, and impossible to hear any stuttering. Now, shrink it even more, because now you can use the other end of the binoculars, and bring the past before, and the future free together now … smoothly, easily, flowing together. It is now the present you give yourself."

Dr. Dan suggested that George practice his yo-yo breathing everyday, to go someplace wonderful in his imagination, and imagine his speech smooth and easy.

"Then," said Dr. Dan, "bring it back with you to the present, the present that you give yourself."

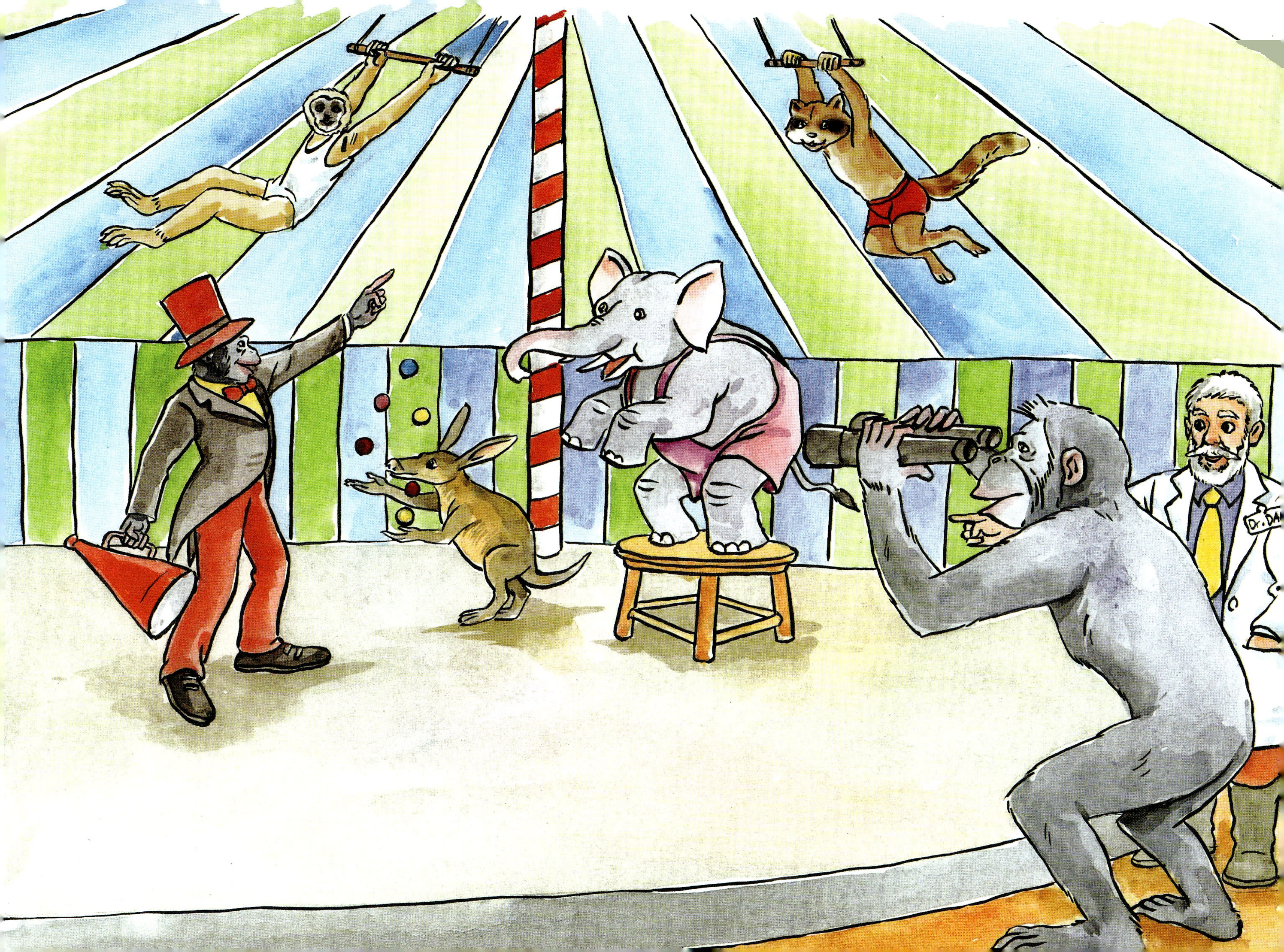

Jud Alpaca

Jud was a cria, a baby alpaca. His family came to the Ashland Zoo from the mountains of Peru. Alpacas are friendly, furry animals who live in large groups called "herds." They eat grass, hay, and oats. Alpacas are related to llamas, but they are only about half their size. When Jud was fully grown, he would be about three feet tall, from his shoulder to the ground.

Like their parents, crias have long, soft, silky hair that can be one of eighteen different colors ranging from whites through browns and blacks. Jud was pure white.

When alpacas get angry or scared, they spit. What made Jud spitting mad was pooping. All the Alpacas in the alpaca area at the Ashland Zoo went to the same place to poop. Jud hated to poop in the same place where all the other alpacas went. When he was a little cria, and his parents were beginning to toilet train him, Jud didn't mind peeing in the poop pile, but no way would he poop there. He decided to just hold his poop inside.

Jud's little belly got so full of poop, it gave him a tummy ache. Then, unexpectedly, the poop came bursting out all over his silky white fur. Jud was just a little cria then, and he didn't understand that it was important to poop almost every day. His bottom got so used to holding in his poop that his brain stopped paying attention to the signal that he needed to go. The little cria would go for days without pooping, then a giant poop would come out at just about any time, any place. It wasn't Jud's fault that he couldn't stop the poops from coming out. In between the giant poops, little squirts came out. Jud couldn't stop those, either. This became a big problem for the little cria. The poop smelled bad, and some of the other alpacas called him "Stinky."

Alpacas are valued for their fur. Like sheep, their fleece can be clipped, and the wool made into coats, hats, and blankets. Nobody wanted Jud's fur because it was smelly and dirty.

Harry Hypno-potamus was Jud's friend. He never called him "Stinky." He told Jud, "You aren't the only one with this problem. It even has a name. It is called *encopresis*. Lonnie Llama used to have this problem, too, until Dr. Dan, our zoo's veterinarian, helped her become the boss of her poops. I'll bet that he could help you, too, so you can learn to control what you never knew you could."

"I do want to be the boss of my poops," the little cria declared.

Jud trotted over to Dr. Dan's office. The veterinarian checked Jud over very carefully.

"I can feel a lot of poop in your belly," he told Jud. "The first thing we need to do is to get all that poop out."

Jud's mom gave him an enema. She put water into Jud's bottom, and it rinsed out the poop. The enema made Jud's tummy ache a little, but it sure felt better afterwards.

Jud went back to see Dr. Dan, and together they worked out a plan. After breakfast and after supper, Jud would go to the alpaca's poop pile and stay there for several minutes. After eating is a good time for poop to come out. Dr. Dan suggested to Jud's mother that she could give the little cria some medicine that would keep his poops nice and soft. Jud would be responsible for washing his bottom and keeping his fur nice and clean. Dr. Dan suggested that Jud keep a calendar of his success. Jud called it his Super Duper Pooper Chart. He put a sticker on the chart every time he went to the poop pile without even being reminded, even if he didn't actually poop. When his bottom stayed clean all day, Jud got another sticker. When he did poop in the alpaca poop pile, he got even more stickers. At first, Jud didn't like being at the pile, but Dr. Dan taught him how to use his imagination to think about fun stuff while he was sitting there.

Dr. Dan told Jud all about his special gatekeeper valve: "Just like everybody else who poops, you have a very special gate-keeping valve. It is the only valve in the world that can tell the difference between a gas, a solid, and a liquid. For years, scientists have been trying to figure out how to make such a wonderful valve, but they haven't succeeded yet. Your body has its own gate-keeping valve, but right now it isn't working."

Dr. Dan told Jud a story about a gatekeeper: "When a vehicle approached the guard house, a light was supposed to go on. The light was a signal to the guard to open the gate. One day, a big tractor trailer truck

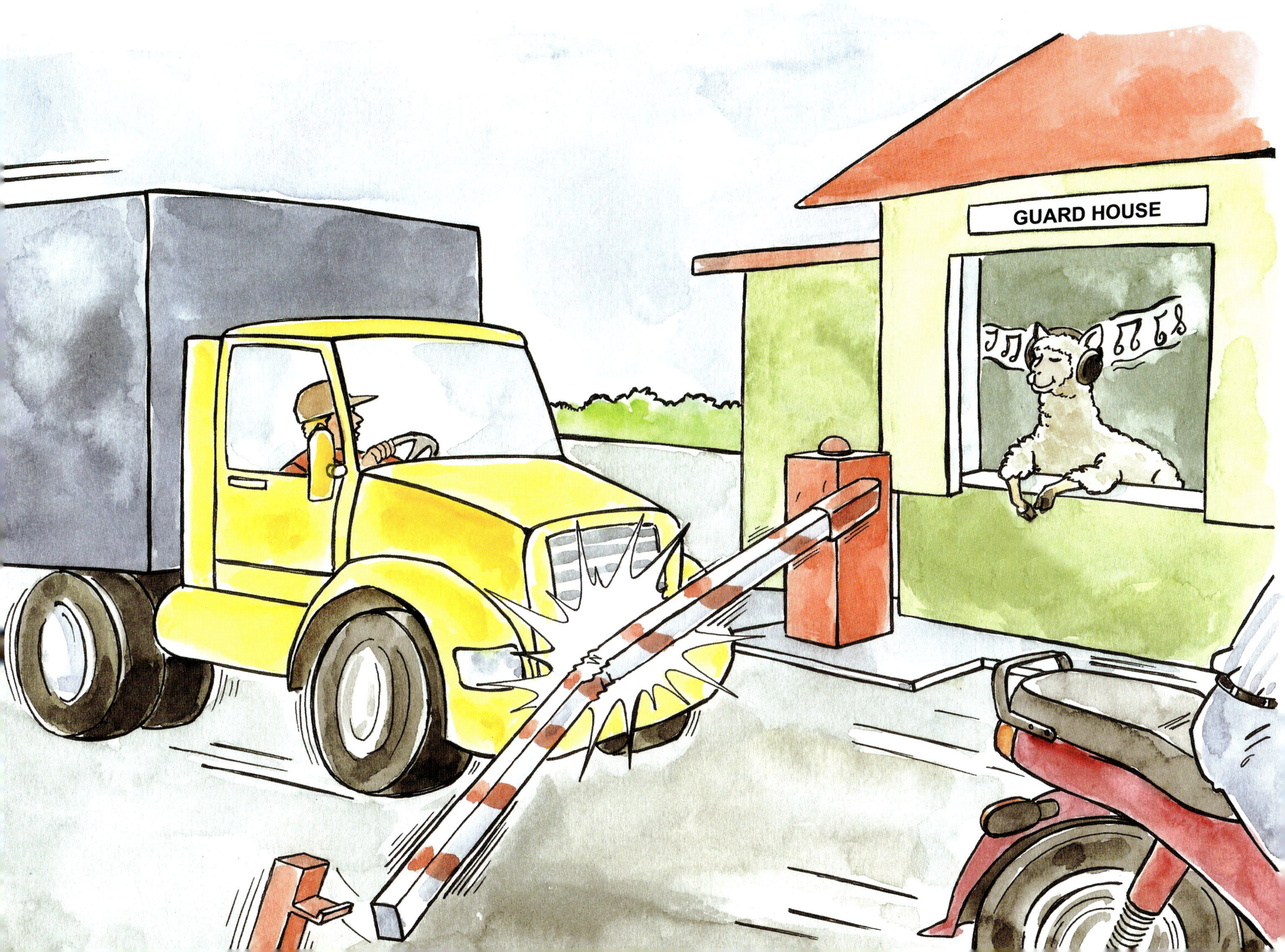
GUARD HOUSE

approached the gate, but the signal light never went on. The tractor trailer truck sounded its horn, but the guard had on headphones so he couldn't hear the sound. He didn't know that the big truck wanted the gate to open so it could pass through easily.

"Traffic started to back up behind the trucks. Then, when the guard wasn't paying attention, several guys on motorcycles snuck around the trucks and slipped under the gate. Then, the big tractor trailer truck was getting so much pressure from behind, it crashed through the gate.

"After the motorcycles snuck through, and the tractor trailer truck crashed through, the gatekeeper's boss knew that the gatekeeper was not doing a good job. The gatekeeper's boss had a choice: he could either fire the gatekeeper and hire someone new, or give him a good talking-to. He could tell the gatekeeper not to wear headphones when he needed to be paying attention.

"The gatekeeper and his boss had a talk. After they talked, the gatekeeper and his boss discovered that the signal light wasn't working. It was not the guard's fault.

"Together, the gatekeeper and his boss developed a plan. First, they cleared away all the traffic that was backed up and waiting to go through the gate. Every morning and every night, the gate would be opened for any vehicles that wanted to pass through. The gate would be kept closed for the rest of the day, but the wiring would be fixed so the signal light could alert the guard when a vehicle wanted to go through. Soon, everything was working smoothly. The boss was so proud of how well the guard was doing that he gave him a special reward."

Jud took the special medicine that his mother gave him to keep his poops soft. Every morning and night, after eating, the cria went to spend a little time where all the other alpacas pooped. Soon Jud was the boss of his poops. His Super Duper Pooper Calendar was full of happy faces. Jud's coat was the whitest, softest, and best-smelling fur of all the alpacas.

Kluft Turkey Vulture and Kahn Quetzal

Kluft was a turkey vulture who lived with his family outside the Ashland Zoo. The vulture's job in nature is an important one, but rather messy. When an animal was hit and killed by a car on the road outside the zoo, Kluft and his family came to get rid of the body. Because they have such a messy job, only a vulture's body is covered with feathers. The vulture's head is bald.

If a predator threatens a turkey vulture, the bird throws up. That throw-up smells so bad, it frightens away the attacker. Kluft got so good at throwing up, it became a habit—something he did really well, without even thinking about it. After a while, whenever Kluft got even a little nervous, he threw up. Soon, nobody wanted to be around him because he was always throwing up.

Kahn was a quetzal, a brilliant green bird with a bright red breast and long tail feathers. Kahn came from a cloud forest in Costa Rica. That's where avocado trees grow high in the mountains. Quetzals eat the fruit of the avocado tree, and swallow the chestnut-sized avocado whole. Their stomachs digest the fruit and throw up the pit. Kahn thought this was gross. He was afraid to eat avocados because he didn't want to throw up.

Kluft threw up all the time, and Kahn was so afraid that he might throw up that he was afraid to eat. Their parents thought that Dr. Dan, the Ashland Zoo's veterinarian, could help.

"Kluft and Kahn's bodies know just the right way to get rid of anything they have eaten that might be unhealthy for them," Dr. Dan told the parents. "Their tummies can warn their brains of danger if the food they have eaten is bad or full of germs. Kluft and Kahn have strong muscles in their wings that help them fly, and they have strong muscles inside their tummies that help them digest food. These muscles know how to work together to help the food go through their bodies in one direction. Sometimes, though, it is important to stop the food from going through their bodies, and bring it up in the opposite direction. Tummy muscles know just how to do that easily and comfortably. Kahn's tummy muscles have forgotten to remember what they knew that they had known—that throwing up is important sometimes. For Kluft, throwing up has become a habit, something he does really well without even thinking about it. Habits can be controlled, though, and hypnosis can help."

Dr. Dan talked with Kluft and Kahn to find out if they really wanted to change, or if that was something their parents had decided.

"I want to stop throwing up all the time," Kluft answered.

"I want to get over being afraid to throw up," said Kahn. "I want to enjoy my food again."

Dr. Dan opened his desk drawer and took out two small chains—two very special chains. Each of these very special chains had a metal ball on the end.

Dr. Dan told the birds, "These are called 'Chevreul pendulums.'"

The veterinarian leaned his elbows on his desk and held a chain between his thumb and pointer finger. He said, "Since birds don't have fingers, would each of you hold one of the pendulums in your beak? You might want to wish to imagine flying high above the trees, gliding easily and peacefully on gentle wind currents."

As Kluft and Kahn soared through the skies in their imagination, Dr. Dan said, "It would be fun to learn how I could talk to your inside brain without either of you having to say anything. When I ask each of you a question, and the answer is 'yes,' the pendulum will begin to move. I'm not sure which way it will move. Perhaps the pendulum will move around in a circle, or perhaps it will swing back and forth, from right to left, and left to right; or, when your inside brain is thinking 'yes,' perhaps the pendulum will move back and forth, from bottom to top, and top to bottom. There is no right way or wrong way. Your inside brain will know the correct way to move the pendulum when you are thinking 'yes.' Without either of you trying to move the pendulum, you can just wait and watch."

Then Dr. Dan asked, "Does Kahn have brilliant green feathers?"

As Kahn thought about the answer, which was "yes," his pendulum began to move slowly from right to left, and back to right again.

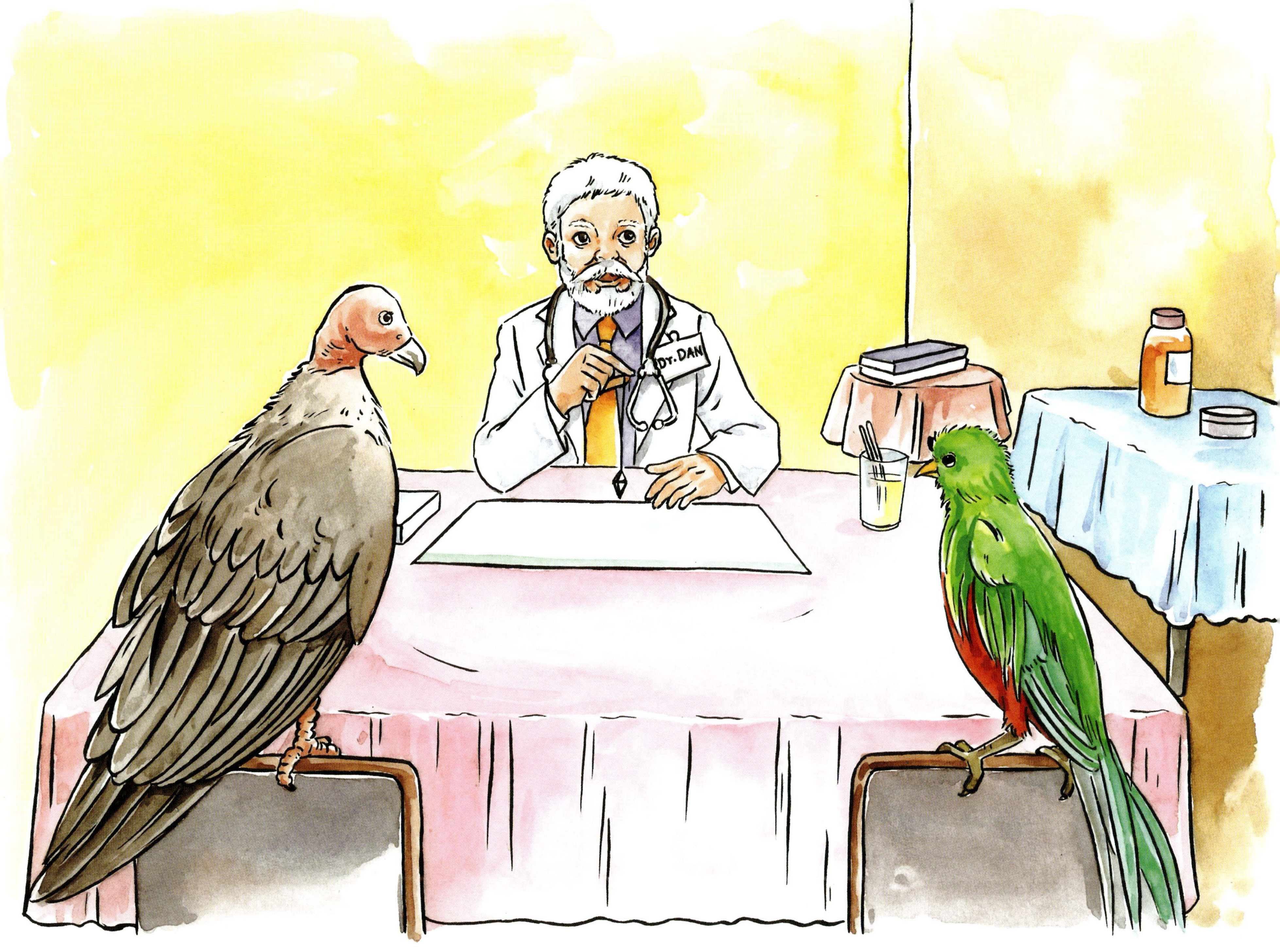
Dr. DAN

"Good," Dr. Dan responded. "If I ask you a question, and the answer is 'yes,' your inside brain will tell me the answer by moving the pendulum back and forth, from right to left.

"Now, as you continue to fly above the trees in your imagination, I'll ask you a question that has a 'no' answer. It will be fun to notice, as you think about the answer 'no,' which way the pendulum will move."

Dr. Dan asked the question: "Do you live in Antarctica at the South Pole?"

Again the pendulum began to move. This time the ball swung in a straight line, up and down, from bottom to top.

"Because your brain never has to give me an answer unless it wants or needs to, the pendulum may move in a different direction if I ask you a question and you are not ready to give me the answer yet."

As Kahn began to think about that, the pendulum began to move again, this time in a circle.

"Excellent!" said Dr. Dan. "If the answer to a question is 'yes', your inside brain will move the pendulum from right to left. If the answer is 'no,' the pendulum will move from bottom to top. If you are not ready to answer the question yet, the pendulum will move in a circle … That's wonderful! Just continue to imagine that you are doing something really fun in your imagination."

Kahn pretended that he was flying under the canopy of the cloud forest.

Dr. Dan asked the beautiful bird, "Are you ready to be the boss of your fear of throwing up?" The pendulum began to move back and forth, from right to left—the "yes" answer.

"That's wonderful!" said Dr. Dan.

Then Dr. Dan repeated the same thing with Kluft to find out how the pendulum would move for "yes," for "no," and for "I'm not ready to answer that yet."

Dr. Dan asked Kluft, "Do you want to stop throwing up except when it is necessary?"

The pendulum moved in the direction that Kluft's inner mind had decided was the "I'm-not-ready-to-answer-that-yet" movement.

"Some things you may not want to tell me, and I'd like you not to tell me before you are ready … now … to tell me."

Kluft said, "I thought it would be too difficult to stop. I was afraid that if I tried, I wouldn't be able to do it."

Dr. Dan said, "If you want to stop throwing up all the time, I could teach you hypnosis. With hypnosis, you could learn to control what you never knew you could. Hypnosis is thinking to help yourself, daydreaming on purpose, imagining success so that you can be successful. It has worked very well for others, and it will be interesting to discover how well it works for you. The pendulum will let me know with a 'yes' when you are ready to take that next step."

Kluft's pendulum moved in the "yes" direction.

"That's wonderful," said Dr. Dan. "Great."

Dr. Dan began by teaching Kluft and Kahn belly breathing: "As you take a slow **deep** breath in, feel your belly slowly rise … Then, even slower, **gently** let your breath out … That's right … Very good … Another slow **deep** breath in as you breathe in happy thoughts … then, as you let go of your breath … let go of worried thoughts … Breathe in **calm** … and as you breathe out, feel the **calm** spread from your nose to your toes … Breathe in **comfort** … and as you breathe out, feel the comfort going to all parts of your body … That's right … Excellent … You are very good at this. Breathe in and swallow as you feel that **wave of relaxation** go from your mouth to your throat and all the way **down** to your stomach … calm and comfortable, confident and in control. Breathe in that **confidence** … and let go of worries. As you swallow, feel yourself going even **deeper relaxed** … even **more** comfortable … One way only … going **down** … always going **down** … only when necessary changing direction, and only if necessary, coming up easily and comfortably … trusting that your body knows what it needs to do as you remain **so comfortable** and **so relaxed**."

Dr. Dan suggested that Kluft and Kahn practice their belly breathing every day, feeling the happy, comfortable thoughts go all the way into their tummies. Kluft liked practicing in the mornings best. Kahn's favorite time to do his belly breathing was right before bed. He also discovered that it was great to practice just before eating.

Soon, Kluft was in control of the habit he used to have, and Kahn was no longer afraid to get rid of the avocado pit. Dr. Dan knew the Native American Indians were right. They believe that quetzals bring us beauty and joy along with an important message about letting go of things we don't need.

Dr. Dan was very happy that the birds had learned to control what they never knew they could just by learning how to do hypnosis themselves.

Howard Mongoose

Howard was a mongoose who came to the Ashland Zoo from Africa. He had a long, thin body and a pointed face. Although he was only two feet long, Howard was a fierce fighter and very brave. He was also sick. He had a disease called "sickle cell." Some of his red blood cells were not quite round. Instead, they looked like a thin, curved slice of the moon. As Howard's blood flowed through his body, sometimes these crescent-shaped blood cells got bunched up together, especially in his knees and elbows. When this happened, those knees and elbows would hurt.

One morning, when Howard was lying in the warm sun, hoping the pain would go away, along came Harry Hypno-potamus on his way to his mud bath. When he saw Howard, he invited the mongoose to come with him.

"I'd love to," Howard replied, "but my knees hurt and my elbows hurt and all I want to do is lie here in the sun."

"I think I know how you feel," said Harry, "I used to have a lot of bad toothaches. Dr. Dan, the zoo's veterinarian, taught me how to do hypnosis when I had a toothache so that it didn't bother me. I think Dr. Dan can help you to help yourself with your pain."

"That would be great," Howard said, "Let's go see him right now."

Dr. Dan examined Howard very carefully, then he asked, "How would you like to take the 'ouch' out of your pain?"

"I sure would!" Howard shouted.

"Good," said Dr. Dan. "Now, I would like you to do three things: On one, roll your eyes up. On two, take a deep breath in; on three, as you slowly exhale, allow your eyes and your eyelids to close as they move down together, taking you even more deeply relaxed.

"Now," suggested Dr. Dan, "Go someplace wonderful in your imagination."

Howard was a very good musician. Everyone in the zoo loved to gather round the piano when Howard played, so Howard imagined sitting at the piano playing one of his favorite songs. It made him feel good to imagine making beautiful music.

"Play a song *fortissimo*," Dr. Dan suggested. In the language of musicians, *fortissimo* means "very loud." Then Dr. Dan suggested, "Change the music to *forte* (loud) and then *mezzo forte* (not very loud.)"

"Ah," said Howard, "playing the music loud, then soft is a *decrescendo*. I am very good at those."

"Notice how the music goes along smoothly, like a river, and then make the music get **softer** and **softer** as you play **lighter** and **lighter**, growing **less** and **less** loud, becoming *piano* (soft or quiet) and then *pianissimo* (very soft), the lightest of melodies, **gently**, flowing easily, and then just **fading** away ... Now that it has faded away, I wonder what song would feel the most **soothing**?"

Howard played another beautiful song in his imagination. As Howard was playing that song, Dr. Dan told him the story of a very great conductor. A conductor is the person who directs the whole orchestra. He is the boss of all the instruments.

"The music of the orchestra was very beautiful. If one of the instruments was harsh and out of tune, the conductor would ask that instrument, 'Would you play very softly until you can be tuned. That way, the orchestra can still continue to play, and the music will still be beautiful.' "

Dr. Dan suggested, "You might like to make an instrument of healing, and then hear, see, and feel its comfortable sound, how **gentle** and **soft** its tone, the melody flowing smoothly, **soothing** and sweet.

"I wonder how wonderful it will be, each time you remember this flowing melody of healing in your special place of comfort. It is a place you can return to whenever and wherever you want or need to. The melody of healing is always inside you. You are the conductor, the boss of your body."

Howard had learned the flowing melody of his body's song, and it was beautiful.

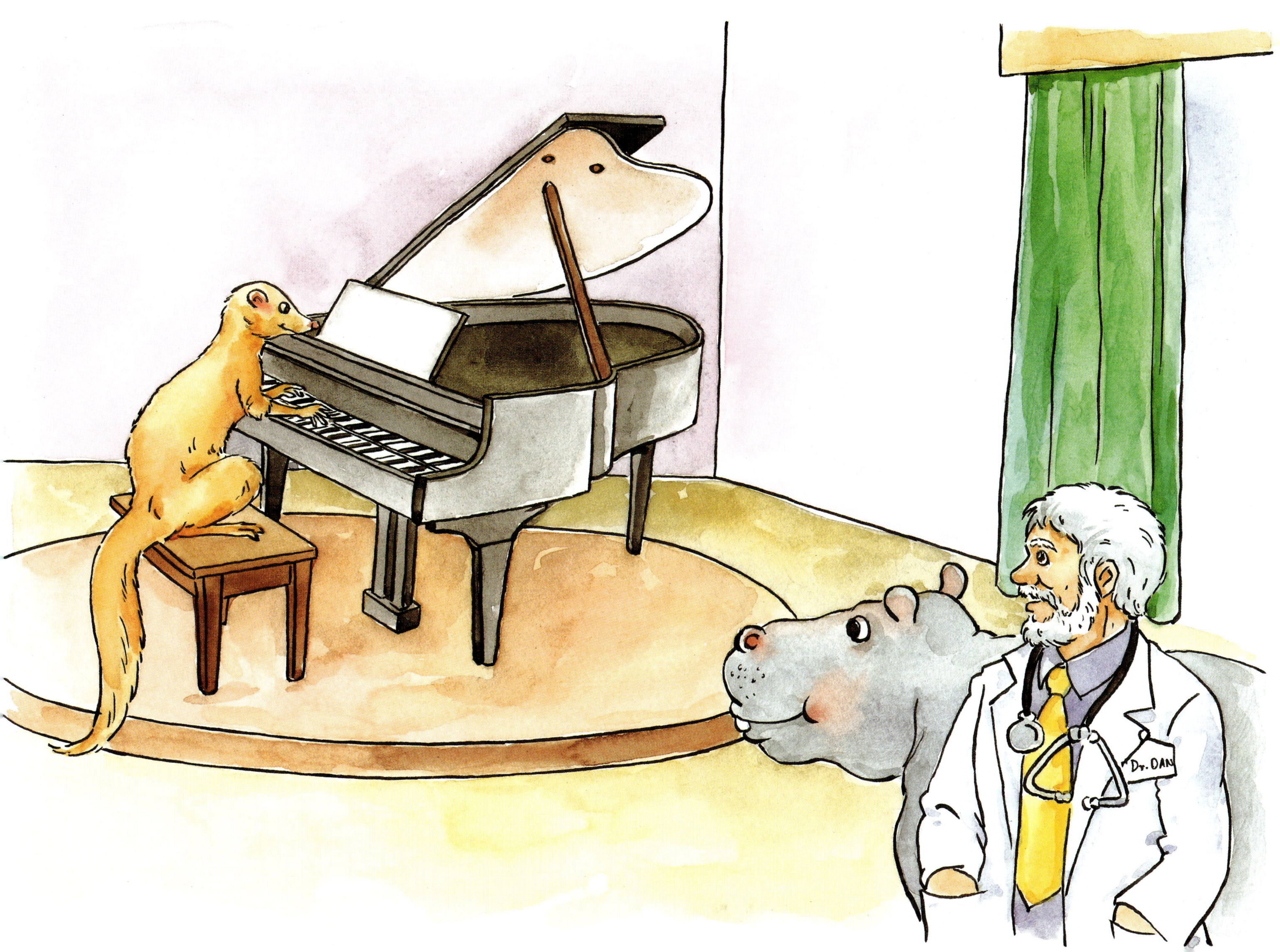
Dr. DAN

Paulker Polar Bear

Paulker was a polar bear who lived at the Ashland Zoo. He was covered with a heavy layer of fat and thick white fur that protected him from the cold. Polar bears come from the Artic. Their white fur helps them to blend in with the ice and snow. Paulker's favorite food was seal, but he would kill and eat almost anything, even it was twice as big as he was.

The other thing that seemed to be twice as big as Paulker was his headaches. The polar bear had a lot of headaches that got in the way of fun things he wanted to do. Those headaches bothered Paulker so much, he decided to get help from Dr. Dan. He was the veterinarian who took care of the animals at the zoo.

Dr. Dan checked Paulker very carefully, then he asked, "What do you already know how to do when you get a headache?"

"I don't know how to do anything," Paulker declared.

"You don't always have a headache, do you?" said Dr. Dan. "Some part of you already knows how to make it go away. What things do you like to do when you don't have a headache?"

"I like to find a chunk of ice and float through the water on it."

"Great," remarked Dr. Dan. "Imagine that you are doing that right now. Hmmmmmm … Floating in the cool water … Feel the waves **rocking** you **gently** back and forth … That's right, the gentle rhythm of the water … rocking … **soothing** … gently **comforting** … both comforting and **comfortable** … **comforting** and comfortable. Breathe in that comfort, and as you breathe out, spread that **comfort** through your body. That's right, breathing in the **comfort**, and sending it to all parts of your body as you breathe out. You may begin to notice that, each time you let go of a breath, almost magically, you let go of tightness and muscle tension. That's good. You are doing this very well.

"As you are floating in your ocean of comfort, ask your head what would be the most soothing right now. What would take the hurt out of that headache?

You **may** wish to take a vacation in your imagination, and leave the headache behind, or you **may** wish to change the pounding to just a gentle tapping. You **may** want to move the headache to a small little spot on your toe where it won't need to bother you. Whatever you decide to do, you **will** feel much more comfortable."

"I think I would like to turn the headache into fish food," said Paulker.

He imagined the headache as a loaf of bread. He pulled off pieces of the loaf bit by bit and fed it to the fish. He could see the headache he used to have going away as the loaf of bread got smaller and smaller, then disappeared entirely.

"That worked great!" exclaimed Paulker.

Dr. Dan nodded and said, "Notice that, somewhere inside your body, you have a comfort meter. It hasn't been working properly lately, but you have all the tools in your tool belt that you need to fix it. So go ahead and do that now."

Paulker imagined using his tools to fix the comfort meter so that it could be turned way up from little to lots to lots more to way more comfort. That felt good: way more comfort.

"Ahhhh," said Dr. Dan, "that does sound good. Take a moment now to picture yourself in the future without those headaches. The future is the present you give yourself now. See it happening, and enjoy that feeling right now."

Paulker remembered all the fun stuff he used to do before the headaches got in the way. Not having headaches was going to be great. If he did have a little one, he could turn it into fish food. And he had all the tools in his tool belt to crank that comfort meter all the way up to way more comfort.

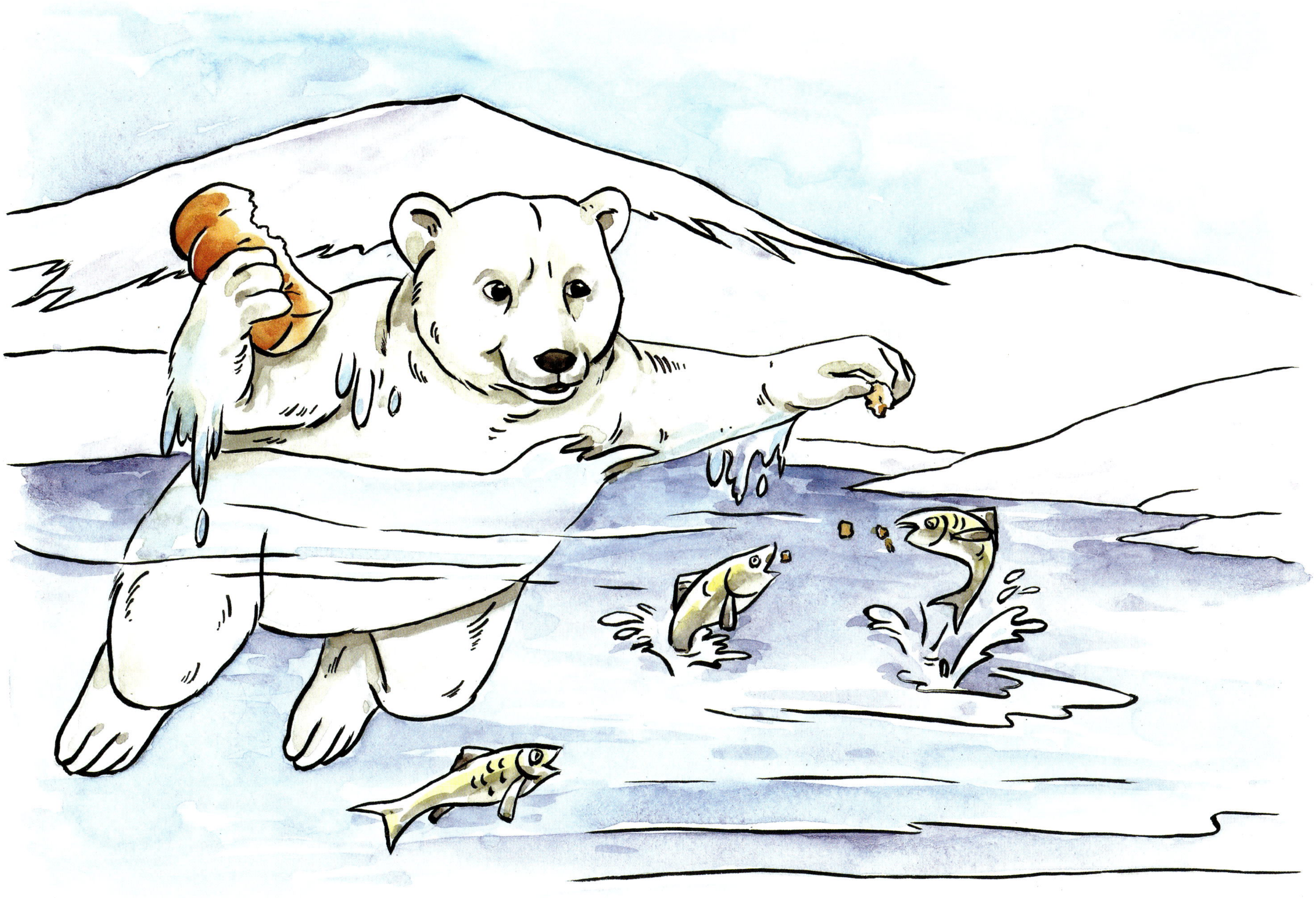

Goldie Lion

Goldie was a lion. She came with her parents from Africa to live at the Ashland Zoo. Goldie's fur was a beautiful golden brown, and that is how she got her name.

Goldie was very proud of her parents because they were very important lions with very important jobs to do. Her father was the king of the jungle, and her mother was the leader of her pride. (A pride is a group of female lions and their young who live and hunt together.)

Goldie's mother and father were very busy lions with many responsibilities. Everyone expected a lot from them. They had to travel a lot, and they always seemed to be working or going to meetings.

"You are our golden treasure," Goldie's father used to tell her.

Goldie didn't feel that way at all. She felt more like a lost treasure. The little lion felt that sometimes her parents were so busy, they forgot all about her. She felt small and unimportant—not like a treasure at all.

When the pride went on a hunt to get food, Goldie felt that she wasn't a very good hunter, that she just got in the way. She worked very hard in school, hoping that her parents would notice how good she was, but she didn't think they ever did.

Goldie began to have tummy aches. They bothered her a lot when she got up in the morning. Sometimes Goldie missed school or going on a hunt, and she got to stay home. At other times, Goldie would go to school, and her stomach would begin to hurt, and her mother had to come and get her. Soon, it seemed that Goldie's stomach was hurting most of the time. Those stomach aches began to get in the way of her having fun with her friends, and it got harder for Goldie to learn her lessons, both on the hunt and in school.

Goldie's mother was worried. She took the little lion to see Dr. Dan, the Ashland Zoo's veterinarian. Dr. Dan checked Goldie over very carefully.

He said, "Your mind and your body are connected, and they talk together all the time. Do you remember the last time your tummy growled? It was sending a message to your brain that you were hungry, and your tummy wanted to be fed. All day long, your brain also sends messages to your body. I'll show you how that works. Hold your paw like this, with your thumb and pointing finger making a circle. I am going to try to break the circle, but don't let me do it."

Dr. Dan used his fingers to try to break open the circle. After some effort, he finally opened the circle.

"Now," he said, "make the circle again, and while your thumb and pointing finger are in a circle, think about something sad, or something that bothers or worries you."

Goldie thought about her tummy aches and her feeling of not being very important. Then, Dr. Dan tried to open the circle made by her thumb and finger. Without any effort at all, he easily opened up the circle. It seemed that all of Goldie's strength had drained away.

"Hmmmmm," mused Dr. Dan. "Now, make the circle again, and think about good things: what a good friend you are, how strong you are."

As Goldie thought about good things, she felt new strength. Sure enough, this time, when Dr. Dan tried to open the circle, her paw was strong and powerful.

"Ahhhh!" said Dr. Dan. "Just by changing what you were thinking about, you changed your muscles. I wonder, when you have those worried, sad thoughts in your head, what messages your brain sends to your tummy, and how that makes your tummy feel.

"I wonder why your body was having those tummy aches," said Dr. Dan. "I wonder what it was trying to tell you, and if it would be alright to tell you in a different way. Perhaps you would like to talk to the tummy ache you used to have and ask it."

Goldie had never talked to the tummy ache before. When she did, she discovered that most of those upset tummies came when she was feeling very small and unimportant.

Dr. Dan told Goldie about the leaf cutter ants that live in the rainforest.

"Leaf cutter ants are farmers. Two million of them live together in one colony. They grow just one crop—a fungus that they eat. They don't eat the leaves they cut; they carry them back to the colony to feed the fungus. A leaf cutter ant can lift thirty times its own weight. That would be like me carrying a bulldozer on my shoulders. They are very strong, and they do very important work.

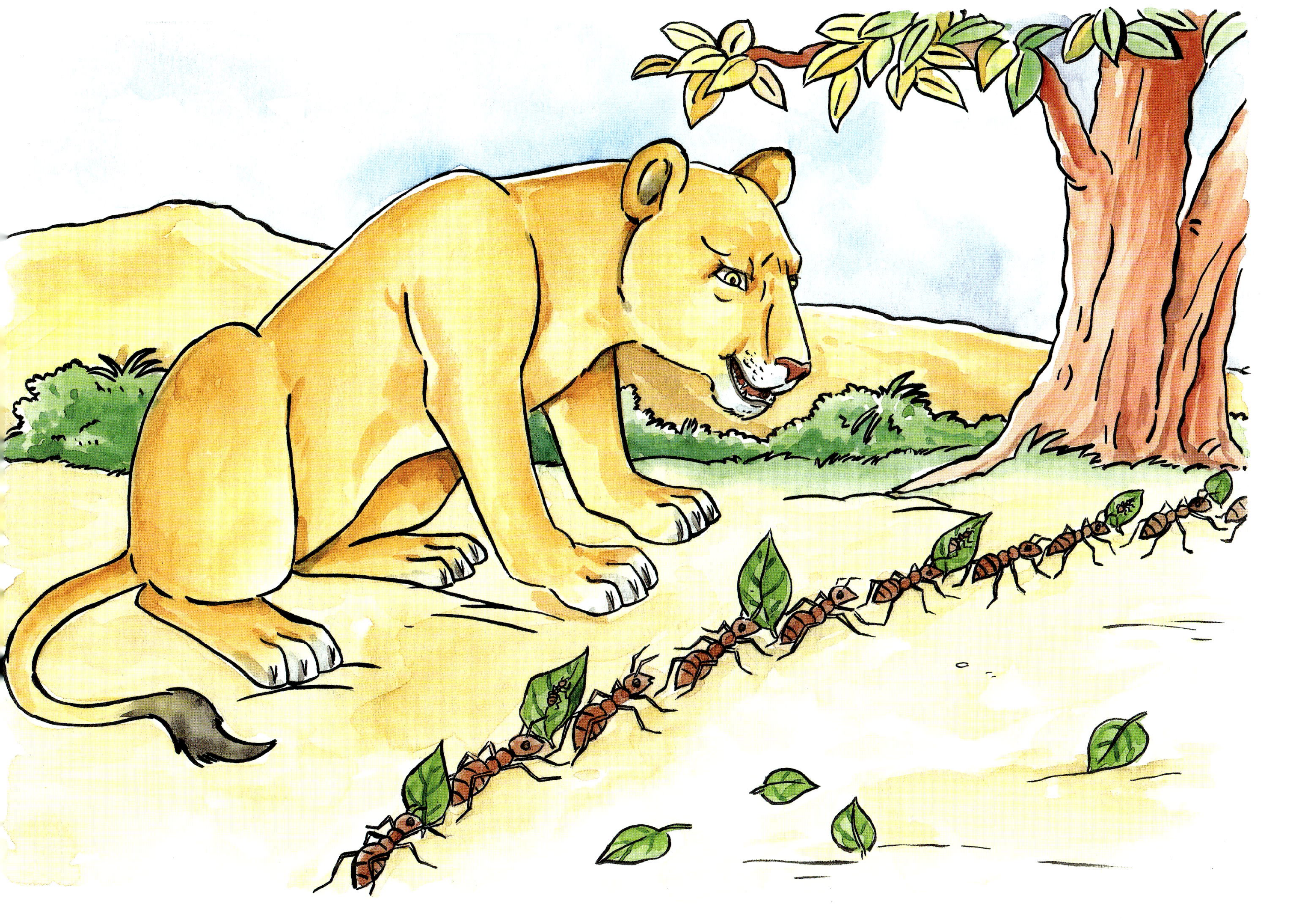

"Some people think the mother, who is called the queen, is the most important ant of all. Actually, the really important ones are the tiniest of her children. These are little bitty ants, called 'minima.' They ride on the leaves cut by the other ants. It is the little bitty ants' saliva that begins to break down the leaf so the fungus can grow big enough to feed all the ants in the colony. Although these minima are very small, they are the most important ants in the family."

"Wow," exclaimed Goldie, "that's cool!"

"Would you like to play the imagination game?" asked Dr. Dan.

"What's that?"

"I'll mention something, and you can imagine how it would look, or feel, or sound—maybe even how it would smell or taste."

"That sounds like fun," Goldie replied.

"There is no right or wrong way to play this game. You can do it with your eyes open or shut—whichever way allows you to imagine better, more easily. Imagine a kitten, how soft its fur feels, how cuddly. Notice how the kitten's tongue feels as it licks you.

"See the sun setting, all red and gold, with its promise of a beautiful tomorrow.

"Breathe in the smell of your mom's cooking—so familiar, so safe.

"Taste what she fixed. It's one of your favorites.

"Listen to the sound of your dad's voice as he tells you one of your favorite bedtime stories. Then, climb up into the rocking chair. I'm not sure if you will be by yourself, or in someone's lap, but enjoy the gentle, soothing rocking."

"That feels so nice," said Goldie.

"Good," said Dr. Dan. "Allow that comfort to come in, come inside to fill the place that used to have a tummy ache."

Goldie said, "My tummy feels good."

"You can play the imagination game anytime you want or need to, all by yourself, or even with an imaginary friend," added Dr. Dan.

Goldie was very good at using her imagination. She imagined doing well at school, and not having tummy aches. Soon, she noticed that she didn't have to imagine it happening, because it *was* happening. She felt like an important part of her pride. Hmmmmm … PRIDE … that was a very good name for the feeling she now had inside….filling her tummy and her whole body … PRIDE.

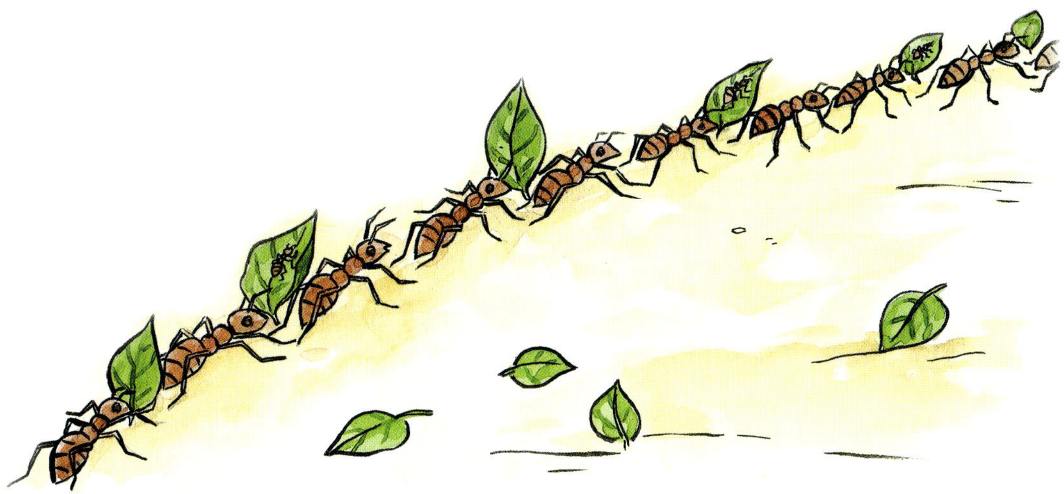

Leora Leopard

Leora was a leopard. Before coming to the Ashland Zoo, Leora lived in South Africa. Her beautiful gold and black fur was soft and silky. She was graceful and smart, and she could run very fast.

The leopard was also very sick. She had a tumor in her brain. The tumor gave her bad headaches and an upset tummy, and it made her feel weak and tired. Leora had to spend a lot of time in bed resting. She also often had to go to the hospital, sometimes for several days. Leora hated the hospital. When she had to stay there, it seemed that someone was always poking her with a needle, or giving her yucky-tasting medicine that made her feel bad. The nights were long and lonely, and she missed her parents.

When Dr. Dan, the Ashland Zoo veterinarian, came to visit the leopard, he brought her a gift: a bottle of bubble liquid. Dr. Dan opened the bottle, dipped the bubble wand into the liquid, and placed the wand in Leora's paw.

"Take a slow breath while you are counting in your mind up to three," said Dr. Dan.

Leora drew in her breath.

"Now," said Dr. Dan, "hold the wand in front of your mouth. Breathe out slowly into the bubble wand while in your mind you are counting up to six."

A whole string of bubbles floated up from the wand. Pretty soon, the room was full of bubbles. Leora noticed, as she continued to breathe in slowly and exhale deeply, as she slowly blew her bubbles, how it made her feel very calm and comfortable.

Dr. Dan suggested, "Anytime that you need to get a poke, you can blow bubbles and blow away any discomfort. I know what a great imagination you have, so if you don't have your bubble wand handy, you can blow bubbles in your imagination. In fact, you can use your imagination to go to a place that's really fun, and leave this place behind."

"How will I get there?" Leora asked.

"Perhaps you would like to ride in one of your bubbles and see where it takes you," answered Dr. Dan.

Leora found the most beautiful bubble, one that was sparkling with a rainbow of colors, and she imagined climbing inside it. Inside the bubble, Leora felt safe and protected. All that hospital stuff could stay outside the bubble. Inside the bubble, Leora brought her favorite stuffed bunny, and she wore her comfiest pajamas.

Her bubble floated on a summer's breeze, and followed a cozy path through the soft clouds, then it stopped for a while at a waterfall. Leora could hear the sound of the water falling over the rocks, and see the sunlight creating rainbows in the mist. Leora's bubble continued on to a playground where it rode the merry-go-round and slid down the curly slide. The bubble stopped at the swings to take a long, lazy ride, gently swinging back and forth … rocking comfortably … so safe … and so comfortable.

The bubble's next stop was in Leora's mother's kitchen. Leora's mother was baking cookies—chocolate chip, Leora's favorite. Leora's bubble was very magical. It could keep out anything that she didn't want bothering her. At the same time, Leora could let in whatever she chose. She filled her bubble with music and the smell of chocolate chip cookies fresh from the oven, then she filled her mouth with the warm, rich, chocolate taste. Mmmmmmm.

Leora had a wonderful trip in her bubble. No one could burst her bubble. If they did, Leora would make another one. She decided that the hospital wasn't so bad as long as she had the bubble of her imagination. With her bubble she took the *dis* out of "disease," and left that on the outside while she climbed into the *ease* on the inside. Then the leopard took the *dis* out of "discomfort," and left that on the outside, too, and filled the inside of her bubble with comfort.

Leora stretched out her beautiful black and gold body and smiled sleepily, safe in the magical bubble that she could create in her imagination any time she chose.

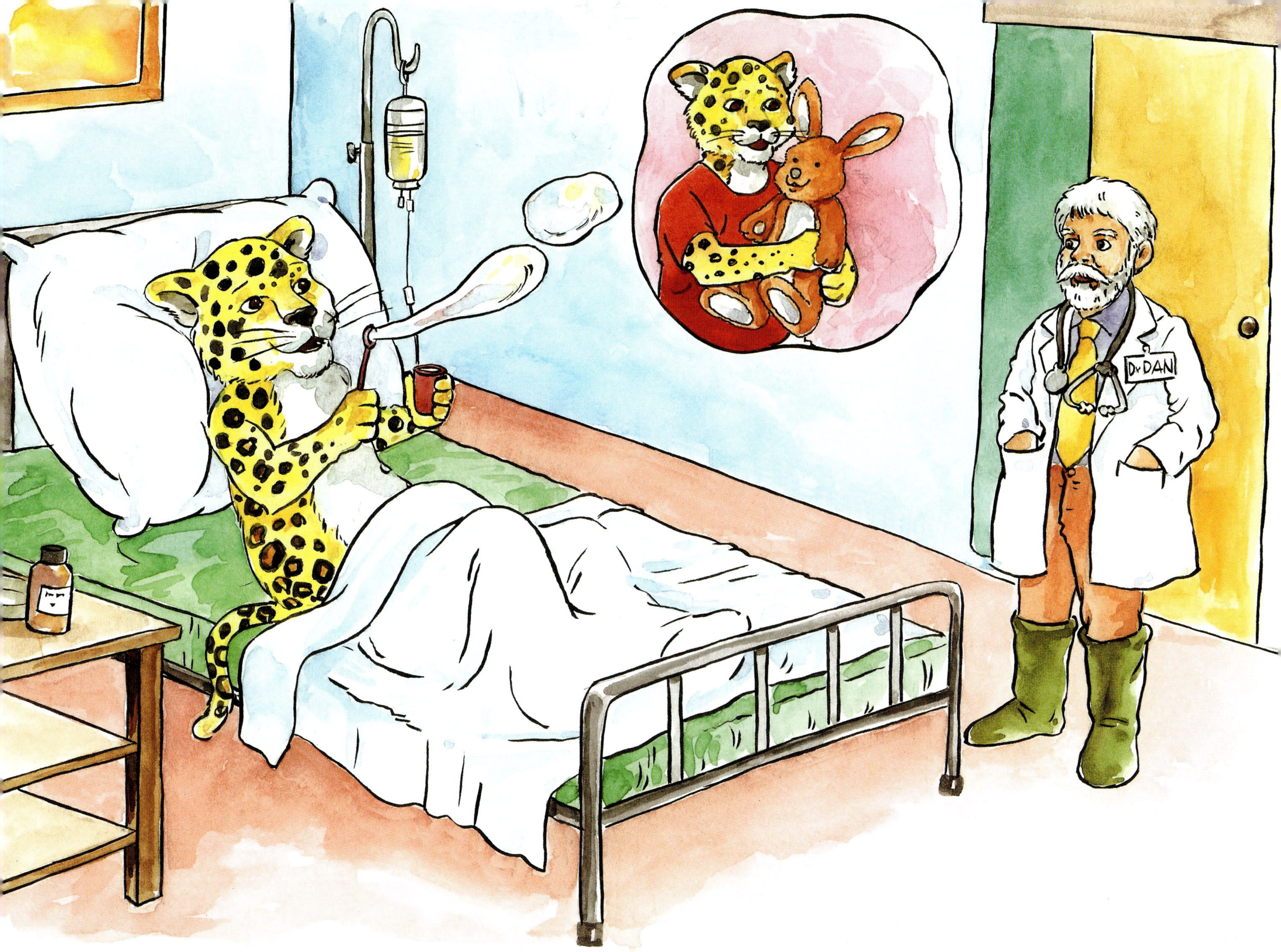
Dr DAN

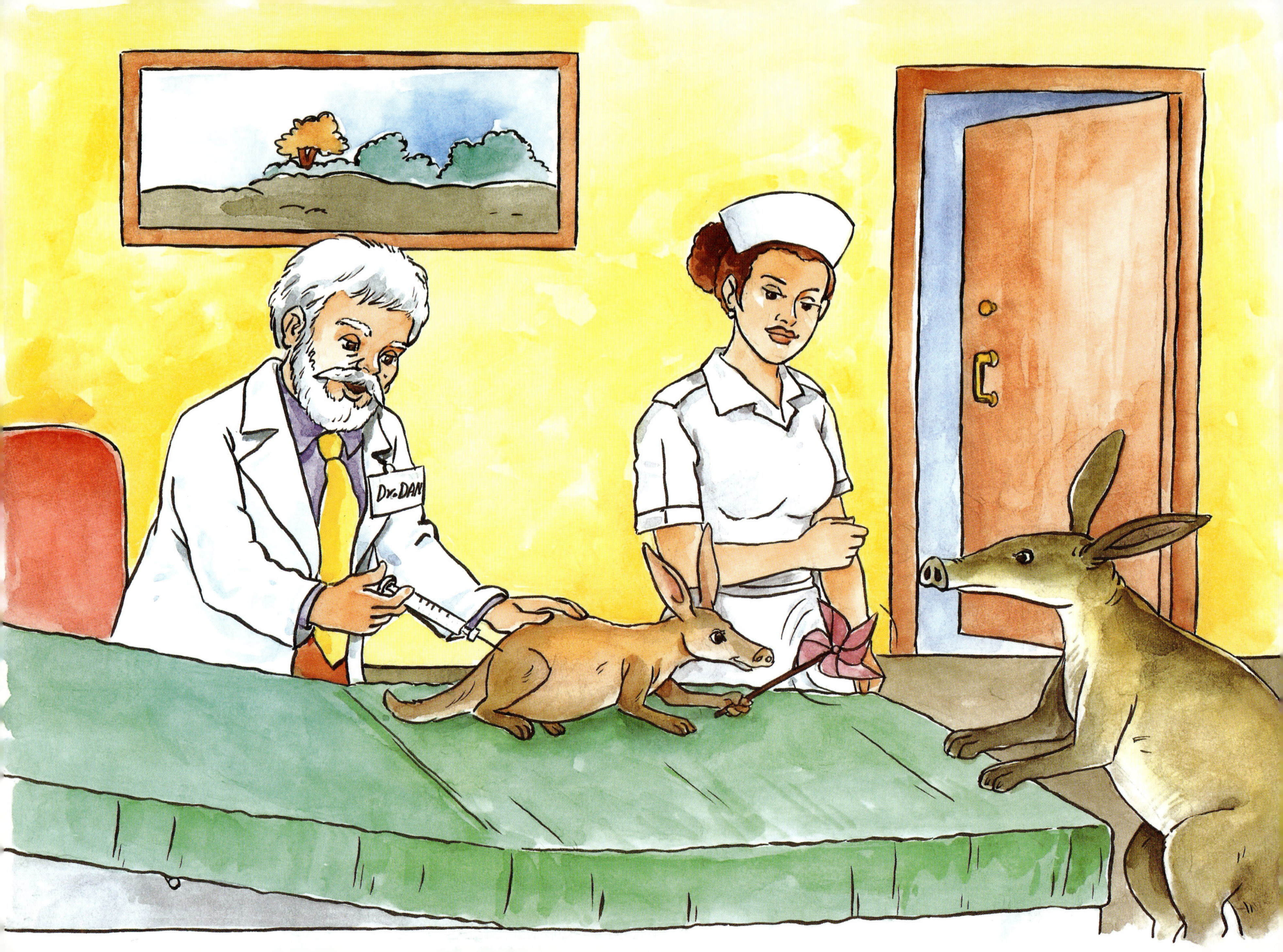
Dr. DAN

Mark Aardvark

Mark was an aardvark. He came to the Ashland Zoo from Africa. Like other aardvarks, Mark had smooth skin with very little hair on it. His ears were big, and his nose and his sticky tongue were long. When fully grown, Mark would be almost six feet from head to bottom.

When the Aardvark was five years old, he was ready to go to kindergarten. Before he started school, Mark needed to have a check-up and some immunizations. His mother made an appointment with Dr. Dan, the Ashland Zoo's veterinarian.

"I don't like going to the doctor," Mark told his mother, "and I'm not sure I want to have a check-up. I'm definitely sure I don't want any shots."

On the morning of his check-up, Mark woke up with a sore throat.

"We'll ask Dr. Dan about that, too," his mother said.

When Mark and his mother arrived at Dr. Dan's office, the nurse named Sally weighed and measured the aardvark to see how much he had grown since his last visit. Next, she wrapped a blood pressure cuff around his arm and pumped it up. The cuff felt like a little hug on his arm.

Dr. Dan did the rest of the check-up.

"I'll show you my special flashlight," the doctor said. "I'll use it for looking into your ears."

As Dr. Dan put his finger on the light, it lit up the finger with a pink glow. The doctor offered the flashlight to Mark and asked, "Would you like to see your finger light up?"

Mark nodded and placed his finger on the light.

"Your finger looks pink because you have nice, healthy blood," said Dr. Dan. "Now, watch this … "

Dr. Dan put the otoscope head on one end of the special flashlight, and lit up a tiny spot on Mark's arm. The spot also looked pink and healthy.

"Which ear would like me to look in it first?" asked Dr. Dan. "Do you have a favorite ear, one you like best? I think they both are cute, so it might be difficult to choose a favorite. Do you have any bunnies in your ear?"

Dr. Dan shined his special light in Mark's ear. "Oh … no bunnies in this ear," he said. "They must have hopped out. I'd better look in your other ear. Nope, none in this ear, either. Do you have any other ears I could look in?"

Mark giggled and shook his head.

"Hmmmmm," said Dr. Dan. "I wonder if bunnies are hiding in your mouth. Open up very wide, and see if you can scare the bunnies out by going Aaahhhh … That was very good, but there are no bunnies in there. However, I did see some very nice teeth. I imagine that you must be very good at brushing them."

Mark nodded. "I brush my teeth two times a day."

"It seems that you have a sore throat today," said Dr. Dan, "so I'll need to find out what kind of germs are making your throat uncomfortable. Your body is very good at fighting off germs, but sometimes you need some special medicine to help your body get rid of them. I will take a throat culture to find out which kind of germs you have in your throat."

From his doctor's bag, Dr. Dan took out a little stick with a tiny ball of cotton on the end. "I am going to tickle your tonsils with this cotton swab," he said. "I wonder if your tonsils will be ticklish. The tickling doesn't hurt, but you might make a funny face like this … "

Dr. Dan stuck out his tongue and made a very silly face. "Now," he said, "let me see your best silly face."

Mark stuck out his tongue and made a goofy face while Dr. Dan gently touched the back of the aardvark's throat with the cotton swab.

"That was a great goofy face!" remarked Dr. Dan.

Mark made another silly face.

Dr. Dan did a special test on the cotton swab. Afterward, he told Mark, "Don't worry, you won't need any special medicine for your throat. Your body already knows how to make it get better."

"Next," said Dr. Dan, "I am going to listen to your heart with my stethoscope. Where did you put your heart last? Where does your heart live?"

Mark shrugged.

"I guess that means I need to look for it," remarked the veterinarian. He laid his stethoscope against Mark's elbow, then he shook his head "Nope it is not there. Maybe it is over here."

Mark began to giggle as Dr. Dan put his stethoscope on the aardvark's knee.

"No," said Dr. Dan, "it isn't there, either."

Finally, Dr. Dan put the stethoscope on Mark's chest and smiled. "Here it is! It sounds like a very healthy heart. What do you do to keep your heart so healthy?"

"I eat good, healthy food," Mark answered.

"That's good," said Dr. Dan. "Exercise is important, too."

"Exercise is fun!" said Mark. "I do that every day."

"That's wonderful," said Dr. Dan. "Now, please take some very big breaths, like this, through your mouth."

Dr. Dan took a very deep breath, then Mark breathed in and out as Dr. Dan listened to his lungs.

Dr. Dan said, "You are very good at breathing. Have you been breathing for a long time? Do you practice breathing a lot?"

Mark grinned and nodded "yes."

"That's why you are so good at it!" said Dr. Dan. "I'll bet that you even know how to breathe when you are sleeping! Notice how each time you breathe out, your muscles feel even more comfortable. That's right. I am going to feel your belly now, so take one of those nice, big breaths, and notice how, as you let go of the breath, your tummy muscles get nice and soft and relaxed. That's right. Very good … Hhhmmmm … Is this ants I feel, right here? What did you have for lunch?"

Mark nodded in surprise, "I did have ants!"

"Now, I am going to listen to your stomach and see if it will talk to me. Sometimes it even growls!" Dr. Dan said as he placed his stethoscope on Mark's tummy.

"Next," said Dr. Dan, "please sit up on the edge of this special table."

Mark hopped up on the long leather table, and Dr. Dan asked him to move his leg.

"It will be interesting to watch how your body knows just what to do without your even thinking about it," said Dr. Dan.

Gently, the veterinarian tapped on Mark's knee with a special rubber hammer that he called a "kneeknocker." Mark's leg moved as if by itself.

"Good!" said Dr. Dan. "You have very good reflexes. That means if you stepped on something sharp, like a pricker bush, your foot would know how to jump off the bush even before your brain told you why you needed to get off. Please jump down so I can see how nice and straight your back is growing."

Dr. Dan examined Mark's back and asked him to bend forward to touch his toes.

"That's wonderful! You are growing just right."

Dr. Dan took some things out of a box and laid them on a table, then he asked Mark, "Would you please walk over to that table and bring me back the green circle? Good, thank you. Now, would you walk over to the table on your tiptoes and bring back the blue triangle? Good. This time, please walk over on your heels and bring me the yellow square. Good. Hop on one foot. Next, switch feet and hop on the other foot."

"This is fun!" said Mark.

"You are very good at hopping," remarked Dr. Dan. Then he said, "There are still a few things we will do to make sure you are all ready for kindergarten. We are going to test your hearing to find out what good ears you have. You will get to wear head phones, and you'll hear little noises in the headphones like this: Hmmm, Hmmmm, Hmmmm … You will need to tell me when you hear the sounds. After that, you will get to look into a machine where you will see pictures of different things—perhaps a car or a house—and you will tell me what you see."

Mark thought that the hearing and vision test was like playing a really fun game.

"Now," said Dr. Dan, "we just have a few more things to do to get you all ready for kindergarten. First, I need to get a little drop of blood from your finger so that we can do a little test. That test will tell us if you are eating enough good foods, and making enough healthy red blood cells. Then, we have to put some medicine into your arm. It may feel like a little poke."

"Will it hurt?" asked Mark.

"Only as much as you want it to, and you didn't want it to, did you? I didn't think so. Perhaps you would like to blow away any discomfort so that the pokes don't need to bother you," said Dr. Dan. "I wonder which would be more fun for you—blowing bubbles, or blowing in a pinwheel?"

"I'd like to blow in a pinwheel," answered Mark.

Dr. Dan produced a very special pinwheel. It was musical. As Mark blew the pinwheel around and around, the pinwheel played a tune. Dr. Dan was right. Mark didn't let the pokes bother him. He was too busy having fun blowing in the pinwheel.

Mark couldn't wait to tell his friend Harry all about his visit with Dr. Dan. When the check-up was all done, Dr. Dan blew up a long, thin balloon. He gave it a couple of twists and made it into a balloon animal for Mark to take home.

Dr. Dan reminded Mark, "Be sure to feel very proud of how well you did at your check-up, and with your shots."

Mark shrugged his shoulders and grinned. "No problem," he told Dr. Dan. "I actually had a lot of fun."

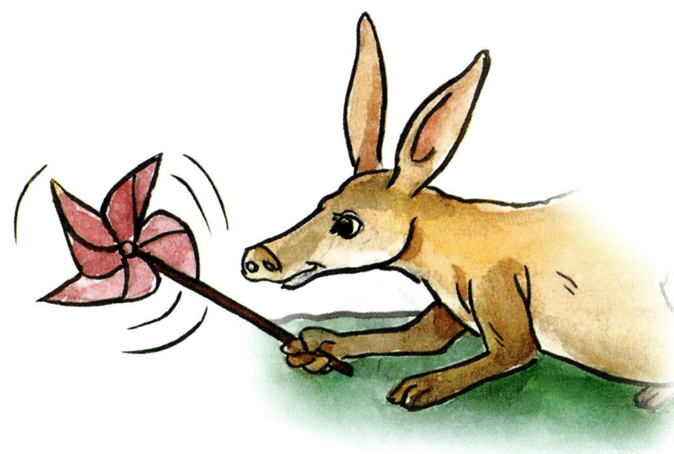

Some of the techniques used in this story were learned in the video, *Imaginative Medicine*, by Laurence Sugarman, MD. It is available through Crown House Publishing.

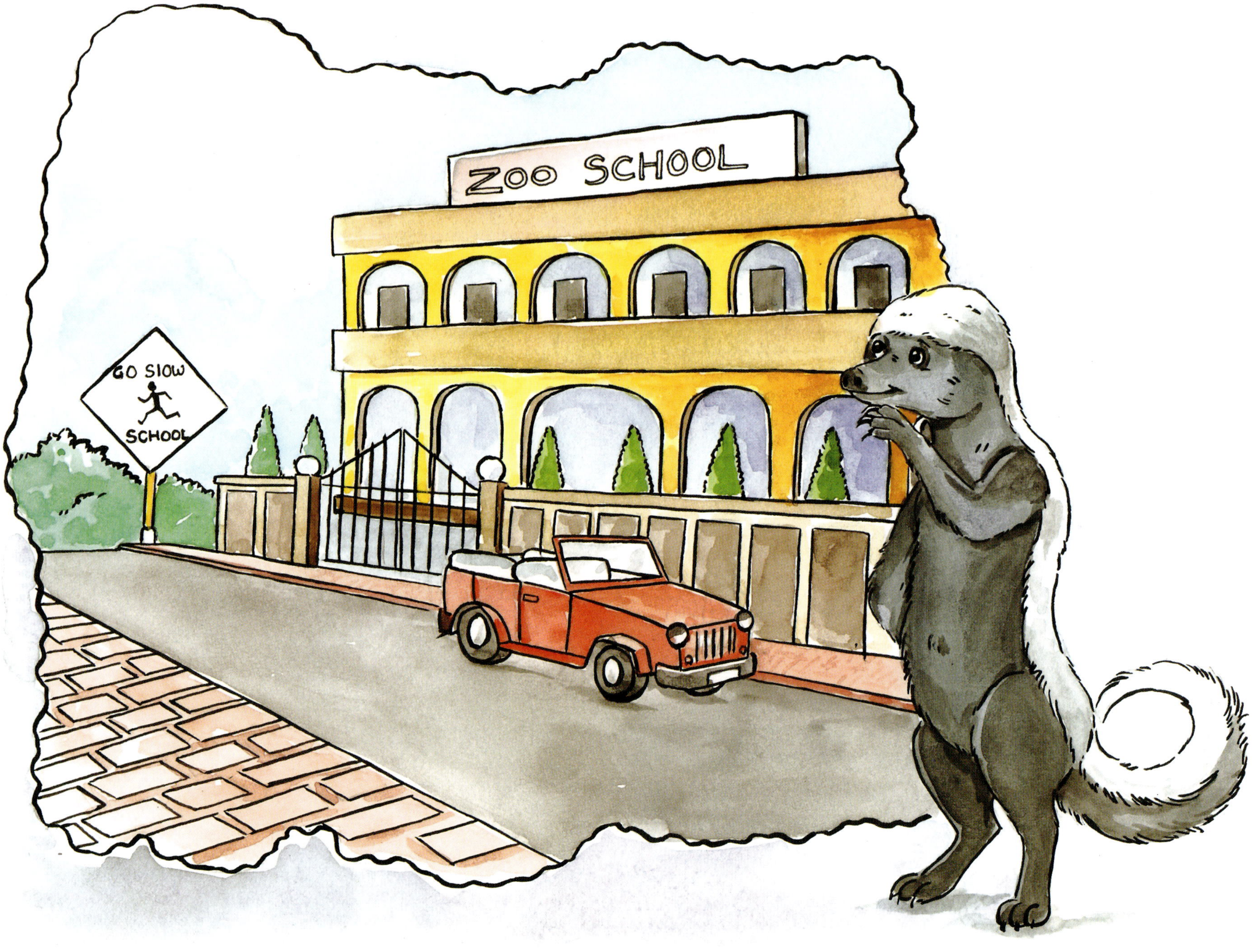
ZOO SCHOOL
GO SlOW
SCHOOL

Raz Ratel

Raz was a ratel. He came with his family from India. The ratels are members of the weasel family. Like their cousins, the badgers, ratels often spend the night digging tunnels. In fact, ratels are often called "honey badgers."

Like his other cousins, the skunks, Raz had a silver stripe that ran down his back from the top of his head to his bushy tail. His tummy was black. If an intruder entered the Ratel's home, Raz would squirt them with his skunk-like scent glands.

Ratels are very busy at night. They spend their days resting in burrows underneath the ground. Sometimes ratels dig their own homes, and sometimes they take over the tunnels built by aardvarks. Raz preferred to dig, and he could dig incredibly fast. In fact, everything that Raz did was fast. He had trouble slowing down and taking his time.

When Raz played hide and seek with his friends, he was great at seeking and finding, but not very good at the hiding part. Oh, he was good at finding a great hiding spot, but he had trouble holding still and being quiet. His moving around always gave him away to whoever was "it."

Sitting still, listening, and paying attention were not things that Raz did best. That was a problem for him when he went to school. Even though the ratel was very smart, he had difficulty concentrating. It was hard for Raz to do his lessons and his homework. He always seemed to be getting into trouble, and he spent a lot of time in the principal's office.

One day, Mr. Thomson, the principal of the Ashland Zoo School, came to see Raz's mother. He told Mrs. Ratel, "I'm worried about Raz. He has a difficult time staying in his seat at school and following his teacher's instructions. Sometimes Raz does things without even thinking about whether or not it is a good choice, and that gets him into trouble. Perhaps Dr. Dan, the zoo's veterinarian, can help."

"I don't know why I have to go to the doctor's! I'm not even sick," said Raz.

"But you do have trouble with your school work," said his mother.

The next evening, they went to see Dr. Dan.

"You know," said Dr. Dan, "every so often I take my car in for tune-ups. These are like check-ups, and they keep my car running really well."

"I like cars," said Raz.

"If you were a car, what kind of car would you like to be?" asked Dr. Dan.

Raz said, "I'd like to be a jeep. They are fast, fun cars, and they can go anywhere."

"Then let's pretend that you are a jeep," said Dr. Dan. "I am going to check your engine and see how you are running."

Dr. Dan checked Raz over very carefully, then he said, "You are a great jeep. Your engine runs just fine. You can climb very fast up hills and over obstacles and sand dunes. You can even go up the rocky slopes of a mountain. However, there are a couple of adjustments that we need to make with your steering wheel and brakes.

"It is great that your jeep can go really fast, but sometimes it is good to go slow so you won't miss important stuff. For example, you might miss the road signs that give directions.

"Have you ever noticed the speed limit signs on the road near your school that tell everyone to slow down? The signs say: 'School. Go Slow.' So it is important to get your brakes fixed for school."

Dr. Dan continued, "Steering is important too. If your steering doesn't work right, it can take you in a wrong direction, or even cause an accident. This jeep is a great car. We don't want anything bad to happen to it because of a little problem with the steering or the brakes."

Then Dr. Dan said, "Fortunately, we have a little pill that we can put into the gas tank. This pill will fix the brakes and the steering. You need to add it to the tank every day so the jeep will slow down in the school zone. The jeep will still have all the power and speed it needs to climb over boulders and up mountains. However, there will be less danger that it will get into trouble because of bad brakes or steering. The jeep will be able to stay on course much better."

Raz said, “I sure could use one of those pills for my gas tank.”

Dr. Dan wrote out a prescription for the special pill that Raz could put in his gas tank. The following week Mr. Thomson, the principal at the Ashland Zoo School, called Raz’s mother and told her what a good job her son was doing in school. When Raz got home from school, his mother gave him a big hug and a kiss.

“I’m so proud of you!” she said.

Raz smiled with glee. “Yup,” he said. “All I needed was some help with my brakes and my steering.”

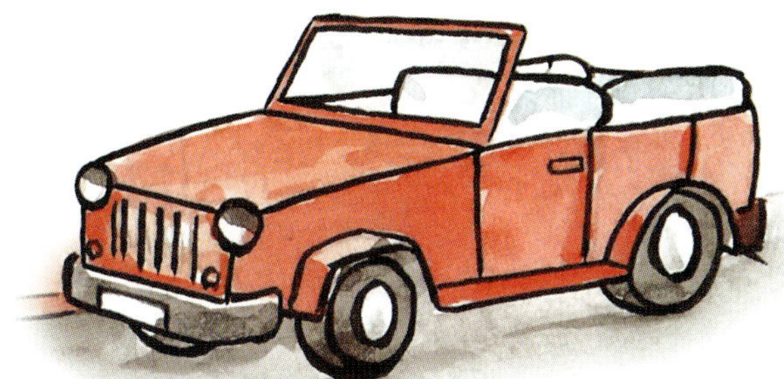

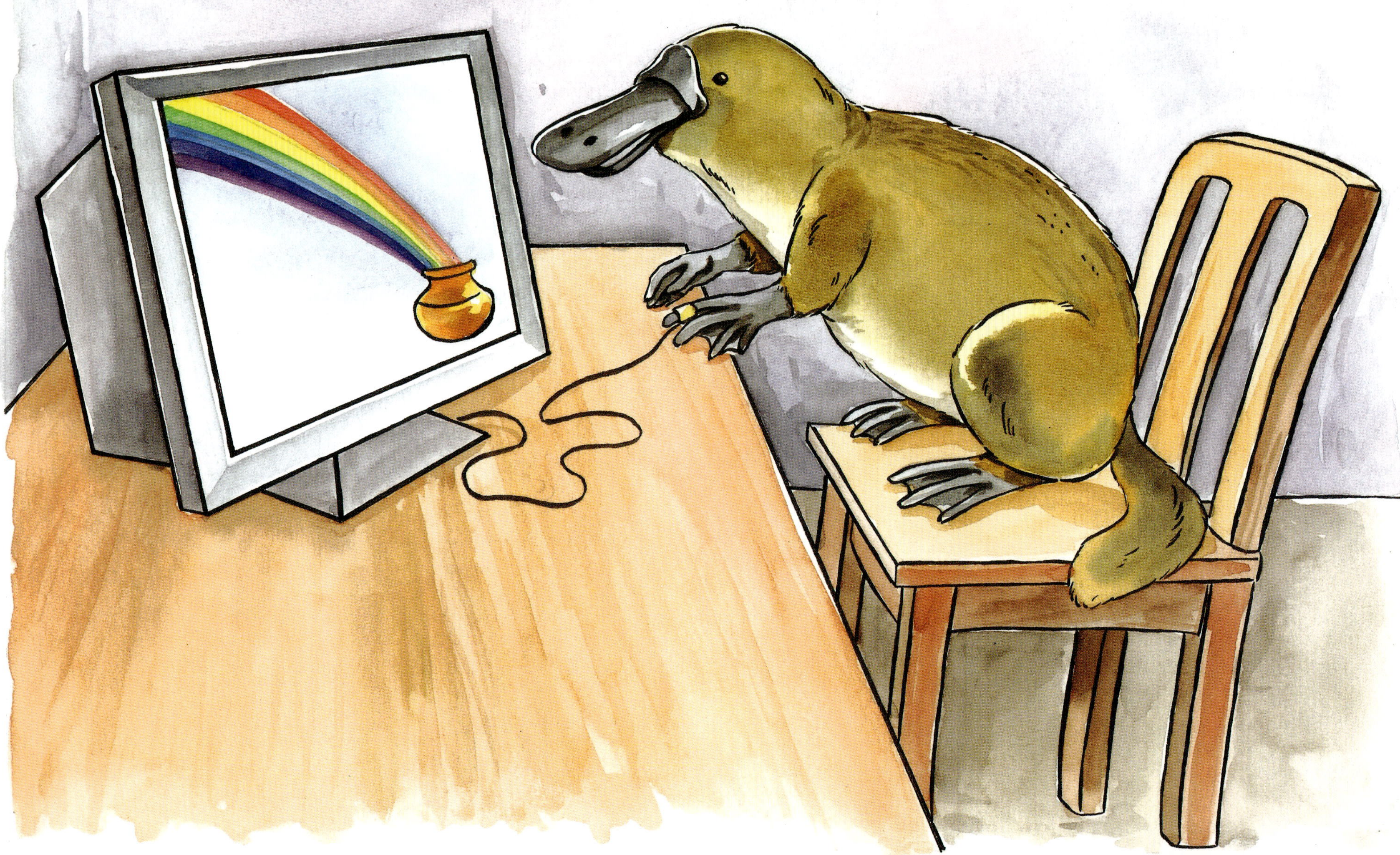

Eric Platypus

Eric was a platypup; that is what a young platypus is sometimes called. He came to the Ashland Zoo from eastern Australia. Even though Eric was a mammal, he was hatched from an egg. His body was wide, flat, and covered with dark brown fur, like a beaver's, but he had a large, rubbery snout that looked like a duck's bill. In fact, platypuses are sometimes called "duckbills."

Eric spent some of his time on land, but mostly he stayed in the water where he liked to eat shrimp and crayfish. He located his prey with special sensors located on his bill. Those sensors could detect electrical fields given off by prey. The process is called "electroreception." A platypus is the only mammal that locates food this way.

Eric would swim underwater, turning his head from side to side, hunting for food. He often got so involved in hunting for crayfish that he sometimes forgot that he needed to come up to the surface for a breath of air. Once, the platypus almost didn't make it up in time, and he came up gasping and choking. Eric worried that it might happen again.

He thought, "I could have been paying better attention, then I would have swum to the surface sooner. I should have been more careful. I coulda. I woulda. I shoulda."

The coulda–woulda–shoulda kept running though the platypus's mind and prevented him from doing anything. As he continued to worry about what he could have, would have, or should have done, Eric started to worry and be afraid of silly little things. Finally, he went to see Dr. Dan, the Ashland Zoo's veterinarian.

"Perhaps you would like to meet Tim," Dr. Dan suggested. "Tim is a special doctor who uses both hypnosis and biofeedback to help others help themselves."

Eric swam over to meet Dr. Tim, who gave Eric a book called *Be the Boss of Your Body*.[1] Tim had written the book with Becky, a nurse practitioner who also helps kids with hypnosis and biofeedback.

After he read the book, Eric went to see Dr. Tim again.

"I liked the book," he said. "It's got a lot of great suggestions that I can really use."

Dr. Tim explained, "When you have too many worries, your body, your mind, and your spirit get out of balance, or rhythm, with each other. Stretch out and get **comfortable** … Imagine a wave of comfort and relaxation going from your nose to your toes … allowing all of your muscles to feel soft and loose … Breathe in through your nose as you silently count to three … and slowly **let go** of your breath through your mouth as you count to five … Feel your belly button rise as you breathe in … and sink **deeper down** … as you breathe out."

Eric noticed that just by changing his breathing, he was feeling more comfortable and relaxed.

"Biofeedback is like a video game for your body," Dr. Tim explained. The biofeedback game that I use is called 'Freeze Framer.'"

Dr. Tim put a little sensor on Eric's webbed front foot. The sensor picked up little electrical impulses from Eric's heart.

"Hey!" Eric exclaimed, "That's how I catch crayfish—by making use of the electrical impulses I receive."

"Now you can make use of electrical impulses in a new and fun way," said Dr. Tim. "The machine will receive electrical impulses from your heart. You will see on the computer screen how good you are at affecting your body and heart rhythms just by letting go of some of your worries and thinking about fun stuff instead."

As Eric began to relax, a beautiful rainbow started to appear on the computer screen. It reached all the way to a golden pot. As Eric relaxed more and more, forgetting about his worries and stress, the pot began to fill with more gold. Whenever Eric let a coulda–woulda–shoulda back into his thoughts, the rainbow began to disappear.

Eric decided to change his thinking from coulda–woulda–shoulda to can do–will do–did do. When his negative thinking changed to positive, the rainbow returned again.

"I like hypnosis and biofeedback," Eric said. "It is like the book that you and Becky wrote."

Dr. Tim nodded. "You can *Be the Boss of Your Body*. And that is true."

1. Culbert, Timothy, and Kajander, Rebecca. *Be the Boss of Your Body.* Minneapolis: Free Spirit Publishing, 2007.

Ran Rhinoceros

Ran was a white rhinoceros. He came to the Ashland Zoo from South Africa. The only land mammals at the zoo who were bigger than Ran were Yapko and Elkins. They were elephants. Ran weighed two and a half tons. He had two horns on his head and a heavily armored body. His hide wasn't really white. When the first English settlers came to South Africa, they heard the Dutch settlers call the rhino "weit". That sounds like "white," but it actually means "wide." The word was used to describe the rhino's mouth which is very wide, and works like a lawn mower to gobble up grass.

Ran had a friend, a bird named "Mesmer." Mesmer was a yellow-billed oxpecker, an African bird with shiny black feathers and a long bill. Mesmer spent a lot of time on Ran's back eating fleas, tics, and flies from the rhino's hide. Ran thought that he was very lucky to have such a good friend, but whenever Mesmer sensed danger, he flew away to safety, leaving Ran all by himself.

The bird began to tease Ran. He would say, "You're so fat and lazy and slow, anybody could beat you in a race."

At first, Ran's feelings were hurt. Then he said to himself, "I'm going to show everybody that I can run fast. I'm going to run in the Ashland Zoo Road Race."

When Ran told Mesmer what he had decided, the oxpecker said, "You will need to begin to train so you will be in shape to run fast. I will be your coach."

With Mesmer riding on his back, Ran waddled to the road and began to run. At first the rhino moved slowly. He needed a lot of space, and he made a lot of noise, but once he got going, Ran discovered that he was a good runner.

As the race day approached, however, Ran started to feel nervous, especially since Mesmer kept telling him, "You gotta run fast, Ran; you gotta do well; you gotta win that race!"

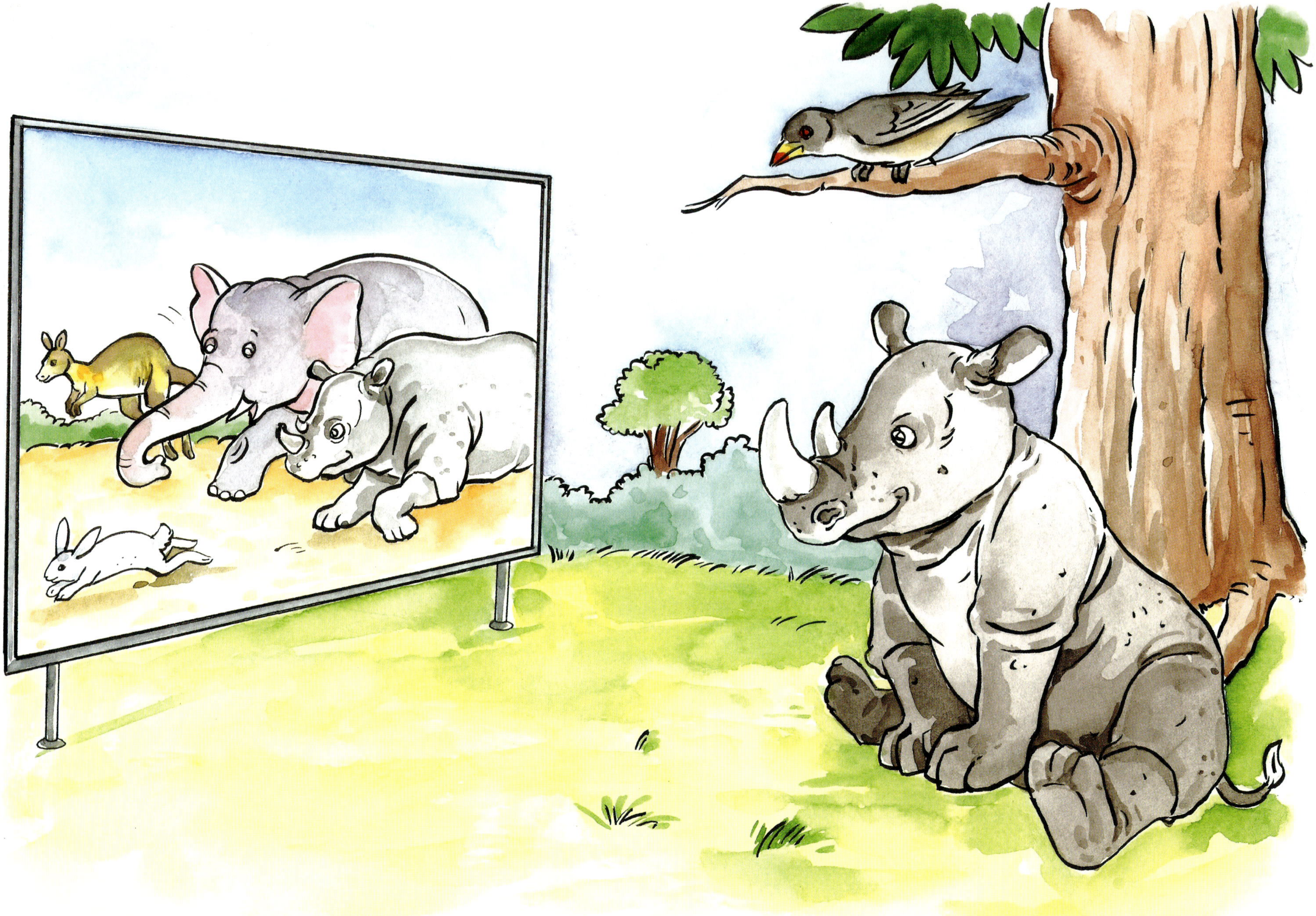

One morning, several days before the race, while Ran was training, he felt like he couldn't catch his breath. The rhinoceros felt scared.

Spiegel Eagle was watching Ran train. Spiegel had asthma, and sometimes he had trouble breathing. He said to Ran, "Why don't you see Dr. Dan, the Ashland Zoo veterinarian, and get help for your breathing."

"That's a good idea," said Ran. And that is what he did.

Dr. Dan examined Ran very carefully and did some tests. After the tests came back, the vet explained to Ran, "You don't have asthma. The muscles in your vocal cords tighten up and make you feel like you can't breathe. Your problem is called 'vocal cord dysfunction.' I can help you learn how to relax your breathing passage—your airway— so that you can calm your breathing yourself."

"That sounds great," said Ran.

Dr. Dan said, "Like Harry the Hypno-potamus, I know that you like taking mud baths, so imagine stepping into a mud puddle with just your feet. Notice how **soothing** and **good** it feels … That's right … Now, go in a bit further as that **comfort** goes higher up your legs, and you go more into **comfort** … Very good. When you are ready, go further into your mud bath as the **relaxation** in your muscles goes up your body. Notice how loose … limp … and at **ease** all your muscles feel … Hmmmmm … **Comfortable** and **relaxed** as you go further. Then, feel that relaxation as it reaches your throat … your throat open, **relaxed** and comfortable … Notice how **easily** and **gently** the air flows in and out. Each breath **relaxes** you even more … **More** comfortable … more **relaxed** with every breath."

"Notice how **calm**, **comfortable**, **confident**, and **in control** you feel. Perhaps you would like to go someplace wonderful in your imagination, a happy place."

Ran knew just the place, and he imagined every detail. He could see it, smell it, and hear all the sounds in his happy place. Imagining that he was there made him feel even more comfortable.

"While you are enjoying that special place in your imagination, notice a movie screen showing a movie of the Ashland Zoo Road Race. See yourself as you would like to look, and feel, and be. Notice your breathing—easy and relaxed. Remembering that you cannot control who wins or loses, you can control doing your best, performing with excellence."

Ran said, “I see Mesmer, and he is pushing me to be first.”

“Ahhh, Mesmer,” said Dr. Dan. “He is the yellow-billed oxpecker who eats your tics and fleas.”

“He’s my best friend,” said Ran.

“Hmmm,” said Dr. Dan. “I think Mesmer eats those insects because he likes the blood inside, and he picks at your wounds so he can get more blood. Mesmer doesn’t do these things because he is your friend. When he senses danger, he doesn’t stick around. If you want to run in the road race, do it because it will be fun; do it because you want to, not because Mesmer wants you to run and be first.”

“You’re right,” said Ran. “I’m going to run for me.”

“Good,” said Dr. Dan. “You have all the **motivation** you need … all the **determination** you need … There is one thing, though … that you still need … that you can receive here today … and … that is … **self-confidence**. Even now, you may feel it increasing. Breathe in that **self-confidence** … and let go of self-doubt. Breathe in **self-esteem** … and let go of tension. When you are ready to come back from your very pleasant daydream, come back, and bring those good feelings, that ‘can-do,’ self-confident attitude back with you.”

“That was cool,” said Ran, “I could see and feel myself running in the race, breathing easily and having fun. I also got a new way of looking at things—like friendships. I know Mesmer, and I thought he was my friend, but that doesn’t mean I have to believe everything he says. I have to believe in myself first.”

“Ahhhh,” said Dr. Dan, “now you know more than you know you know, because now you know what you knew, but didn’t know you knew. Good. Very good.”

And the white rhinoceros gave Dr. Dan a great big wide self-confident grin.

Lankton Lizard

Lankton was a lizard, a very special kind of lizard called a chameleon. Like all the other members of his interesting family, Lankton could change the color of his skin. Some people thought that the chameleon changed colors so he could blend into his surroundings, but that wasn't so. Lankton's color would change if he was scared, or if there was a change in the temperature or light.

Lankton's fast, sticky tongue was as long as his whole body. When he wanted to scare away other male chameleons, he could puff out his throat so that all of him would look bigger.

Lankton was very proud of his skin. He thought it was cool that it could change color, though he liked it best when his skin was green. Then, one day, the chameleon noticed a funny little bump on one of his claws. The bump got bigger and bigger. Lankton didn't like that at all, so he went to see Dr. Dan, the Ashland Zoo's veterinarian.

Dr. Dan examined the bump, and said, "You have a wart. Warts are caused by a tiny, tiny germ called a virus. Warts don't make you sick, they're just annoying little lumpy bumps."

"It looks ugly," Lankton said. "I want it to go away."

Dr. Dan reminded Lankton, "When you get a virus that causes a cold, it doesn't last forever because your body knows how to fight it off so you will feel better. Using your imagination, you can help your body to kill the wart virus."

Dr. Dan continued, "There are also other ways to get rid of warts. They can be cut off, or frozen, or I could put a special medicine on them."

Lankton was quiet, thinking things over. Finally, he said, "The idea I like best is using my own imagination to fight the wart virus."

"Good," said Dr. Dan, "here's what you can do: every night at bedtime, think about those special virus-fighting cells in your body. Imagine that those cells are a small army marching toward the wart, gathering strength as they get closer. Then the army, with its

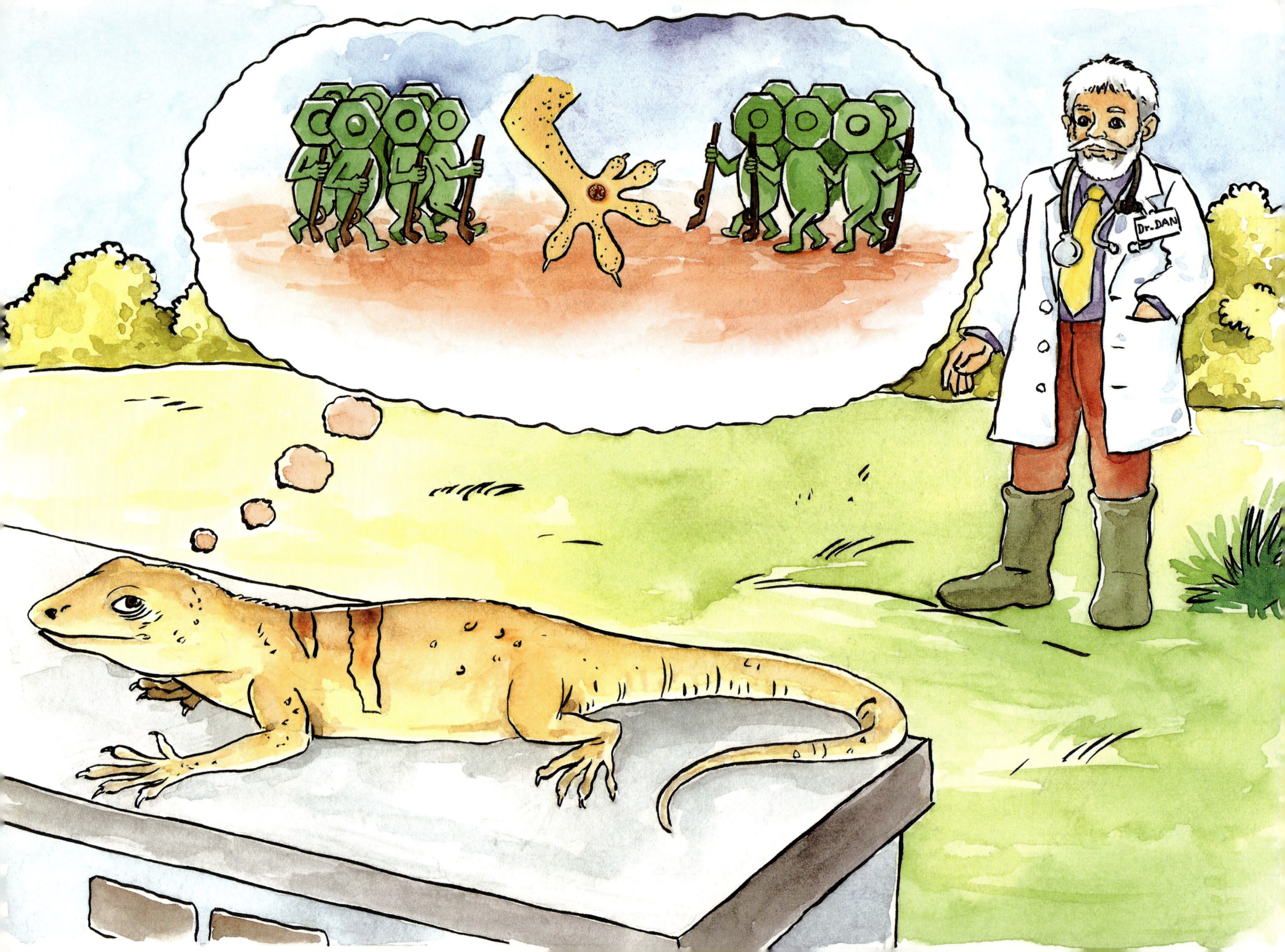
Dr. DAN

powerful weapons, can kill the wart and the virus that caused it. Zing it! Zap it! Destroy it!"

Dr. Dan had already told Lankton that one way of treating warts is by freezing them, so the chameleon decided to imagine also freezing his wart. A polar bear living near the North Pole must have a very cold tongue, Lankton thought, so he imagined the polar bear licking his wart. After that, he imagined freezing the wart again, this time with a penguin kiss.

"An icicle would be another good way to freeze my wart," the lizard thought.

Lankton thought up a lot of other great ideas on how to use his imagination to get rid of the wart. Every night at bedtime, he would picture one of the ways he had imagined to zap his wart. He had fun thinking up a new way almost every night. His favorite was the army of killer cells marching to destroy the virus.

It didn't take very long until the wart just disappeared.

"That's very cool!" Lankton thought. "It's almost as cool as being able to turn green."

"I wonder," said Lankton to himself, "what other cool ways I could use my imagination to help myself. Hmmmmm…mmmm."

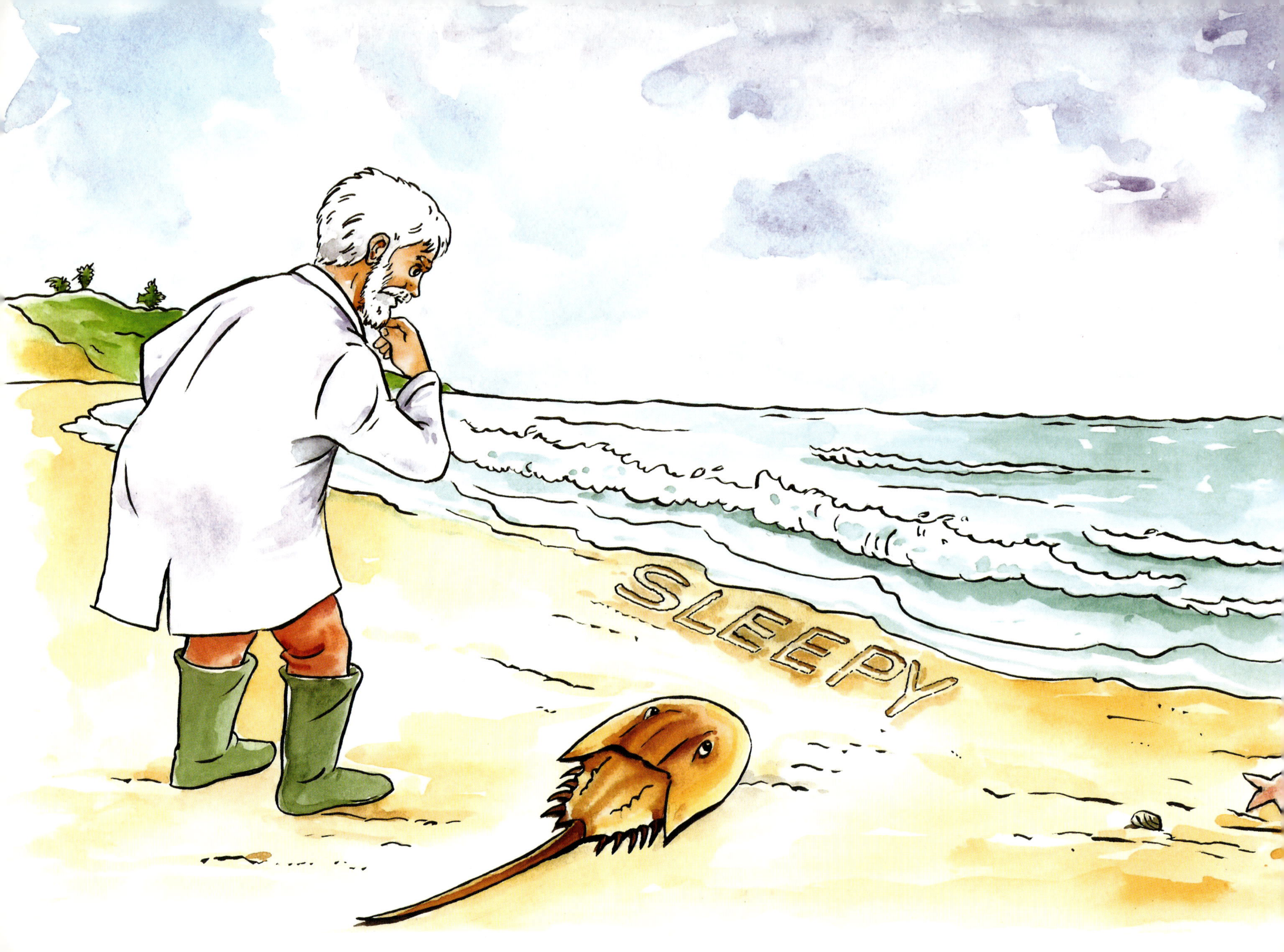
SLEEPY

Carolyn Horseshoe Crab

Carolyn was a horseshoe crab. Actually, horseshoe crabs aren't really crabs at all; they are members of the spider family. Carolyn's ancestors were here on earth 350 million years ago, even before the dinosaurs. She had a helmet-like, armored shell, and a long spiked tail, and she liked to eat worms and clams. Carolyn lived in the salt water along the seashore at the Ashland Zoo.

Carolyn and her relatives have amazing immune systems. That means they are very good at fighting off germs that could make them sick. Scientists have studied and used the blood of horseshoe crabs, which is blue in color, to make sure that medicines for humans are free from germs.

Sometimes, if a big wave came, it would flip Carolyn over on her back. When that happened, the horseshoe crab would use her long, delicate tail to flip herself right side up again. It was important that Carolyn did this quickly. Otherwise, a bird might come to eat her, or she might dry up and die. Dr. Dan, the Ashland Zoo's veterinarian, told all the visitors at the zoo that if they ever saw a horseshoe crab on its back, they should help it by flipping it over, holding not its tail, but the sides of its shell.

Not being able to flip herself right side up was a very big worry for Carolyn. She had a lot of other little worries, too, that got in the way when she was trying to fall asleep. It was hard for Carolyn to shut her eyes to go to sleep. That's because she had lots of eyes. She had seven eyes on the top of her shell, two underneath, near her mouth, and a series of light sensors along her tail.

Dr. Dan was very good at helping everyone discover the magic of their own imaginations so they could help themselves with their problems.

"'Hypnosis' is what I call it," Dr. Dan explained. He suggested, "Each night at bedtime, if you have any worries that are getting in the way of sleep, you can dig a hole in the sand and bury them. The worries can stay there, undisturbed. If you really need any of them, you can dig them up when you wake up, but you might decide to just leave them there in the sand.

Then, with all your worries safely buried in the sand, you can stretch out and think about the feelings that you associate with sleep."

Carolyn thought about feeling snuggly and tired. As she thought about "comfortable" and "sleepy," she began to yawn.

Dr. Dan said, "Imagine writing the word, or drawing a picture of **'snuggly'** in the sand. Then, begin to notice, as you breathe in, a gentle wave comes in, gathering that feeling. As you breathe out … the wave goes back out to sea … and as the next wave comes in, it covers and surrounds you with that **snuggly** feeling … Hmmmm … it feels **so** wonderful and **soothing** … Then, imagine drawing another picture, or writing the word **'tired'** in the sand. As you breathe in, a wave comes in, smoothing the sand … and as you let go of your breath … the wave goes out, and then prepares to return, bringing with it those **tired** feelings … That's right … breathing with the melody of the sea … in and out, growing more **tired** with each wave … more and **more tired** … Now, you may wish to write the word, or draw a picture in the sand, of "**comfort**" … Again, feel the **soothing** wave come in as you breathe in … and out as you breathe out … With your next breath, the wave comes in, bringing in **comfort** … Feel it surround you, both **comforting** and **comfortable**, **gentle** comfort … As you exhale and the wave recedes, feel the comfort flowing through your body … More and **more** comfort … **deeply comfortable** … more and **more** tired.

"I'm not sure," said Dr. Dan, "if you will drift off to **sleep** now, or after writing another word in the sand. Each word you write, or picture you draw, makes you **twice** as **sleepy** as the word before.

"Sketch 'sleepy' in the sand. You may begin to **yawn** as you watch a wave come in and go out, leaving the sand **smooth**. Then a new wave comes in, bringing with it those very **sleepy** feelings, encircling you with sleepiness.

"One after another, the waves coming in with a breath … and going out as you exhale. The waves bringing in those tired, comfortable feelings as the sensations of **sleepiness** get stronger and stronger. Breathing in as the waves come in … and out as the feeling of **comfort** spreads through your body … That's right … Becoming more and more **sleepy** … more and more **comfortable** … Breathing in as the waves come in, and breathing out as the wave goes out. In as the wave covers you in **comfort** … and out as the comfort spreads through your body. Feel the wave covering you with **relaxation**. Notice how each wave takes you **deeper** and deeper **relaxed** … even **more** comfortable, sleepier … drifting **deeper** into comfort."

Dr. Dan said, "You may wish to pretend that you are sleeping, then, pretend that you are not pretending."

As each wave came in, Carolyn became more tired, more comfortable, sleepier and sleepier until she drifted off into a very deep sleep. In the future, anytime Carolyn had worries or thoughts that interfered with sleep, she could bury them in the sand, and then write sleepy, comfortable words in the sand. Then she would feel the deep comfort and relaxation as the waves took that feeling out to sea in order to bring it back in, surrounding and covering Carolyn with comfort and sleep.

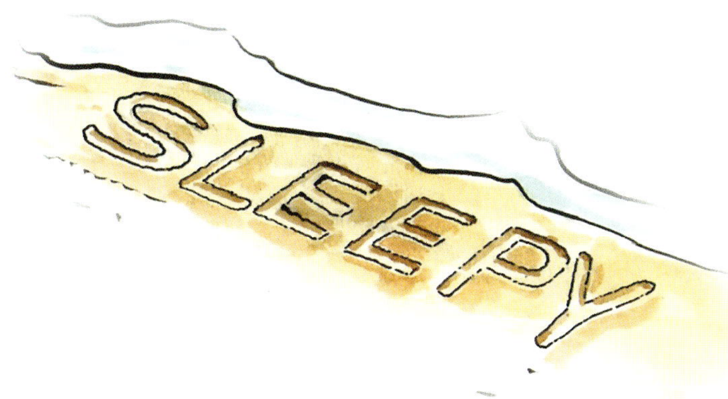

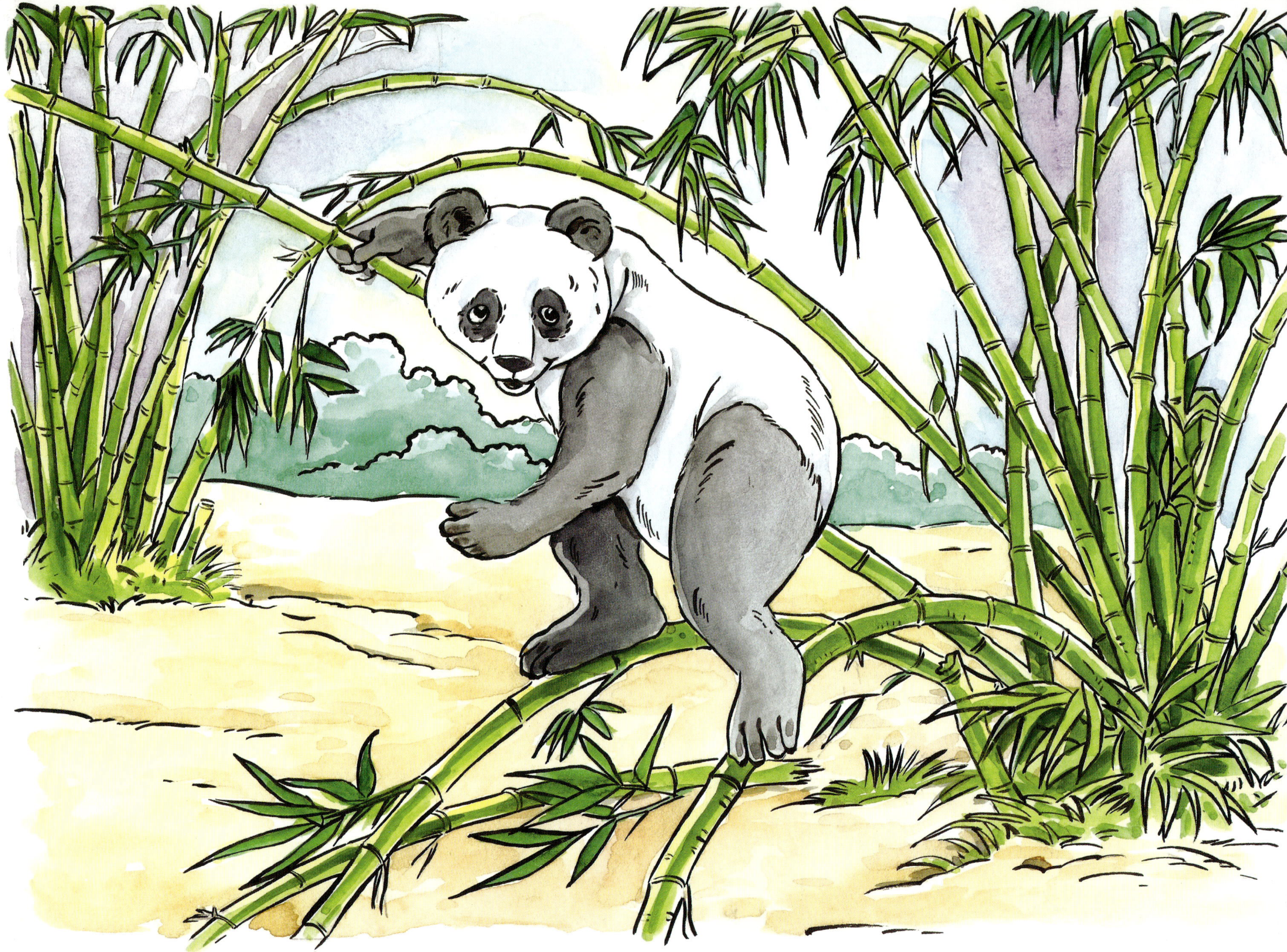

Da-Shih Panda

All of the visitors at the Ashland Zoo loved Da-Shih. He was a panda—a bear-like animal with black fur on his shoulders, legs, ears, and around his eyes. The rest of his fur was white.

Da-Shih came from the rainy mountains of China where there are many bamboo forests. Bamboo was his favorite food, and he had to eats lots of it, because bamboo isn't very nutritious. To survive, a panda needs to eat two different kinds of bamboo, and spend twelve out of every twenty-four hours eating.

In China, pandas are called *Da xiong mao* which means "giant bear cat." They are called that because a panda's eyes look like the eyes of a cat. Unlike bears, pandas always walk on all four legs. They like doing somersaults. In China, the shy panda is a symbol for peace.

When Da-Shih was little, he got lost while he was learning how to explore the bamboo forests. One moment his mother was right there, and the next moment she was gone. Da-Shih couldn't find her. The harder he tried, the more he got lost in the forest. The wind started to blow. Suddenly there was a loud crack, and a big branch came crashing down, just missing the terrified panda. Da-Shih was so scared he began to shake all over. Finally, his mother found the lost panda and gently took him home.

Now Da-Shih lives in the Ashland Zoo. He likes it there, and he has made a lot of friends, but he still misses his home in China. Harry the Hypno-potamus is one of his new best friends.

One day, a few of the zoo workers were trimming branches on some of the trees. There was a loud crack, and a big tree branch came crashing down right near Da-Shih. The panda began to shake all over. He couldn't seem to stop his muscles from twitching and shaking. As the weeks went by, every now and then Da-Shih would start shaking. He didn't really know why. One day, Elgan Elk was passing by, and he saw Da-Shih twitching and shaking. The elk ran to get Dr. Dan.

"Da-Shih is having a seizure," Elgan told the vet. Elgan knew about seizures because he had epilepsy. That happened whenever the electrical messages in Elgan's nervous system got all mixed up, and the elk's body would shake and tremble. Elgan took medicine every day so he wouldn't have seizures.

Dr. Dan did some tests, and he checked Da-Shih all over very carefully. Dr. Dan said, "Da-Shih, you won't have to take medicine to control your seizures like Elgan does. Your shaking is different. I call it 'non-epileptic seizures.' The shaking isn't caused by mixed up electrical signals; they happen when your brain sends unhappy, scared messages to your body without your even realizing it."

Dr. Dan told Da-Shih, "I know what can help you without your having to take medicines: hypnosis. Hypnosis is about thinking to help yourself, daydreaming on purpose. It can help your brain to send good messages to the rest of your body. With hypnosis, you can learn to control what you never knew you could."

Da-Shih began by imagining that he was clinging to a tall bamboo tree that was gently swaying back and forth … back and forth … back and forth … gently rocking. It was so soothing, rocking back and forth. He began to count the rocking. Each number he counted made him feel even more comfortable, even more relaxed, as he rocked back and forth, cradled in comfort. The little panda became so comfortable, it was difficult for him to remember what number came next because he was just so deeply relaxed, as in his imagination he swayed back and forth with the bamboo.

Then Dr. Dan suggested, "Imagine that you are the tree. Feel your roots going down into the ground, giving you **strength** and stability."

The little panda imagined the roots holding and protecting him. He felt the nourishment flow up from the ground through his roots, into the trunk of the tree that was him. That secret, inner strength flowed through him to all parts, all branches, filling every part of the tree. This allowed buds on the tree to burst forth, blossoming with strength and confidence.

Dr. Dan said, "Feel the sun shining, feel its warmth on all your branches. Perhaps the sun might move behind a cloud … a breeze blows … or even rain … cooling rain, bringing its own kind of nourishment to the tree. As night comes, with the stars and the moon, the tree is **safely** rooted to the earth. Feel that **strength** … from its roots through the body, out to all the branches. That's right … breathing in that strength … that **confidence**."

Da-Shih began to practice his hypnosis. Each day, the panda would begin by imagining the gentle swaying, rocking motion of the bamboo, and he noticed how his whole body began to feel comfortable and relaxed. Then, he imagined the tree safely rooted to the ground, and he felt the strength flow right up through his paws to every part of his body. Soon, the twitching and shaking that used to be a problem for Da-Shih was just a memory. He had more important things to do: eat bamboo and pose for pictures for all the visitors at the Ashland Zoo.

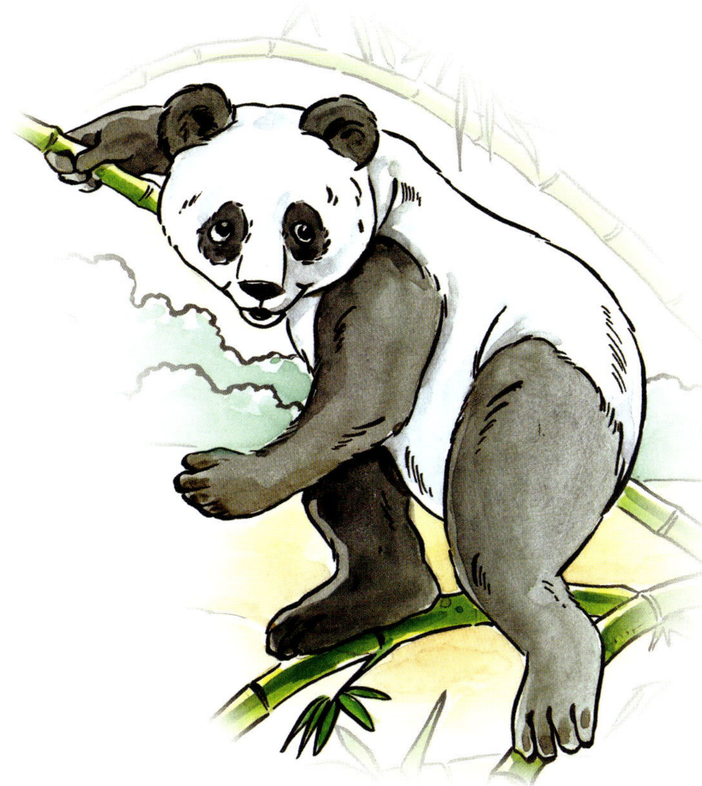

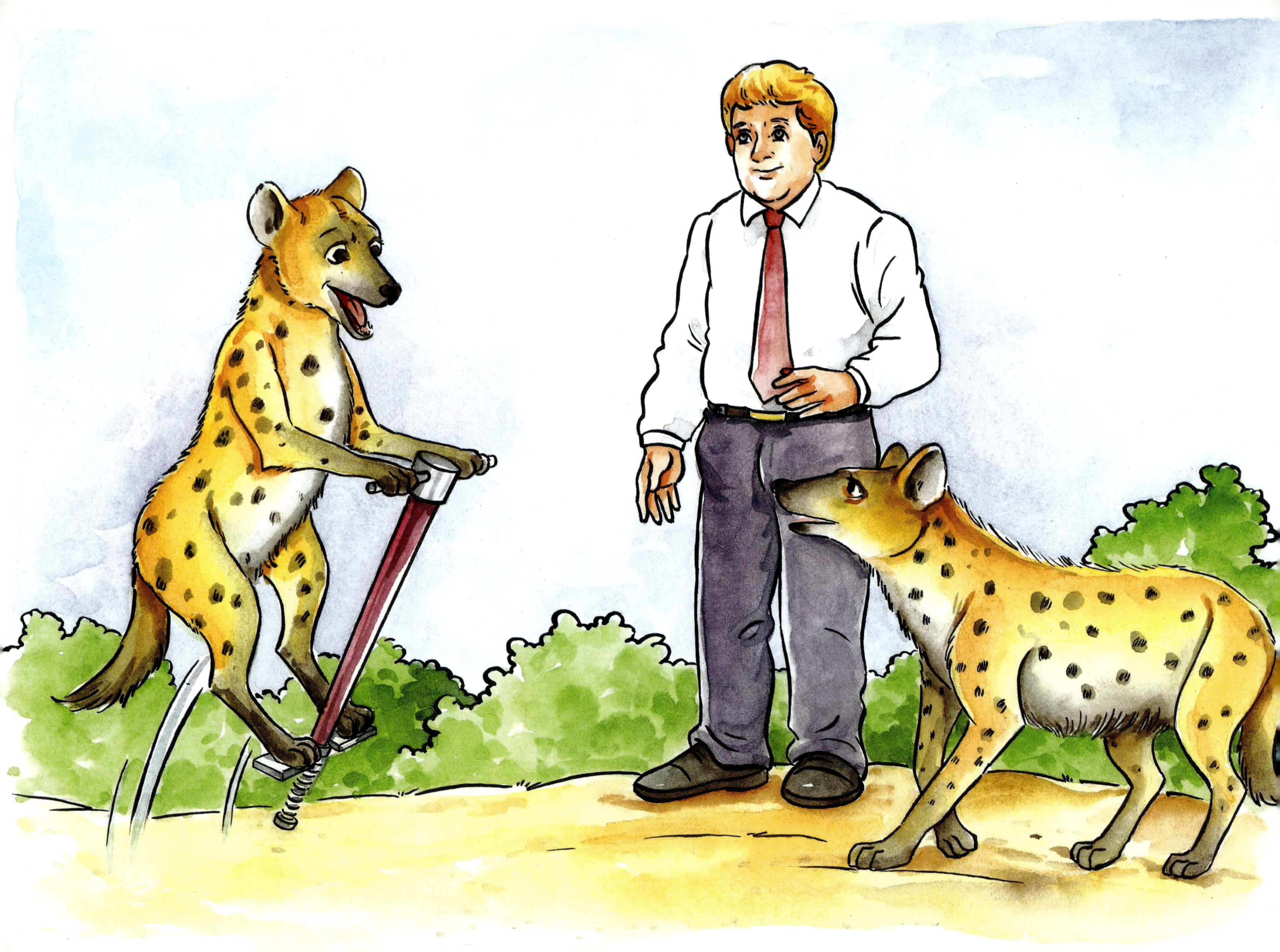

Harvey Hyena

Harvey was a hyena. Like the other hyenas at the Ashland Zoo, Harvey came from Africa.

Hyenas have very strong jaws, large hearts, and front legs that are longer than their back legs. They are very good at cooperating and working together to hunt, and to protect their clan. Hyenas' strength and energy allow them to outrun and exhaust their prey.

People sometimes call hyenas "laughing hyenas" because the noise they make sounds like they are laughing. Harvey, however, didn't feel much like laughing. He always felt sad. When the sun rose in the east, announcing the dawning of a new day, Harvey could not feel glad. Some days, he didn't even want to get out of bed. When the zoo animals all got together to play soccer, Harvey didn't want to play. Sometimes he ate too much because he thought that stuffing himself with food would make him feel better, but it didn't. Instead of a laughing hyena, he felt like a miserable one.

Dr. Moss was one of the zoo's psychologists. He helped animals when they felt sad or depressed. Dr. Moss said that he liked to help others smile at themselves with their own eyes. Harvey had no idea what that meant.

Dr. Moss told Harvey the story of a young hyena named Adam who never felt very happy.

There was an old and very wise hyena named Jack. He asked Adam, an unhappy young hyena, if he would do one new thing each day for a week. The unhappy hyena agreed.

"Today," said the old hyena, "I would like you to do something nice for yourself."

Adam thought about what he would like to do. Finally, he decided to get out his old pogo stick. He had forgotten how much fun it could be to bounce up and down on it. As he continued to jump, the young hyena noticed that a little laugh escaped.

On the second day, the wise old hyena said to Adam, "Today, do something nice for someone else."

That was hard, because the young, unhappy hyena wasn't used to doing nice things for others. Adam thought about his grandfather. The old hyena loved to read, but his eyesight was poor, and he couldn't see well enough to read anymore. Adam decided to read him a story. His grandfather was very pleased, and afterward they shared milk and cookies.

On the next day, the wise hyena instructed Adam, "Do something you have needed to do, but you have put off doing."

Adam knew immediately what that would be. His mother had asked him several times to pick up his toys, but he never felt like doing it. He still didn't feel like doing it, but so far, he had done what Jack had asked him to do, and he liked the way it made him feel. So he picked up his toys. He discovered toys he had forgotten that he had. It was like getting presents on his birthday. Adam also found toys that he had outgrown, and he decided to give those away to his little cousin. Adam felt good about accomplishing that task.

On the fourth day, the wise old hyena said, "Today, do some physical exercise."

Adam thought he would ride his bike, something he hadn't done in a long time. It was a beautiful day, so Adam decided to pack a picnic lunch. He had such a good time that he decided, "Next time, I will invite a friend to join me. That will make it twice as much fun."

The fifth day was for mental exercise. Adam decided to do a puzzle. He liked the way the puzzle pieces fit together to form a picture.

On the sixth day, the wise one said to the young hyena, "Count your blessings and be grateful."

Adam thought about the last few days. He was grateful that he had a pogo stick, and that he was healthy and strong, so he could balance and jump for a long time. Adam thought about his parents, and about being able to spend time with his grandfather and make him happy.

"I guess I am lucky that I have good eyes, and I can read," he said.

Adam remembered all the toys he had, and the fact that he had so many, he could give some away. He also remembered how good it felt to exercise his body and his mind. He had never realized before that he had so many blessings to count.

When the seventh, and final, day of the week arrived, the young hyena wondered what would be next.

Jack, the wise old hyena said, "Today, as you think about the week that has passed, make a plan for the future—for tomorrow, and the day after tomorrow."

Adam had never spent much time thinking about the future, or how he could make tomorrow better than today. He decided to watch what Jack, the old hyena, did during his day.

Jack began his day with exercise. He cleaned out a closet, and he gave several things to someone else who needed them. He did some quiet reading, and then he played a game for fun. As the day was coming to a close, the old hyena took time to be thankful.

When Adam thought about his plan for tomorrow and the next day, he realized that the wise hyena filled every day with six things:

1. He did something nice for himself.
2. He did something nice for someone else.
3. He did something that he needed to do, but had been putting off.
4. He did some physical exercise.
5. He did some mental exercise.
6. He counted his blessings.

Adam started to realize that he was beginning to look forward to the next day and the things he might do. As Adam began to follow the example of his teacher, he noticed he was not so sad anymore. He discovered that he was smiling at himself with his own eyes.

Harvey began to think about the story of Jack and Adam that Dr. Moss had told him. He realized that he was already thinking about tomorrow, and the next day, and a great big smile began to form in his eyes.

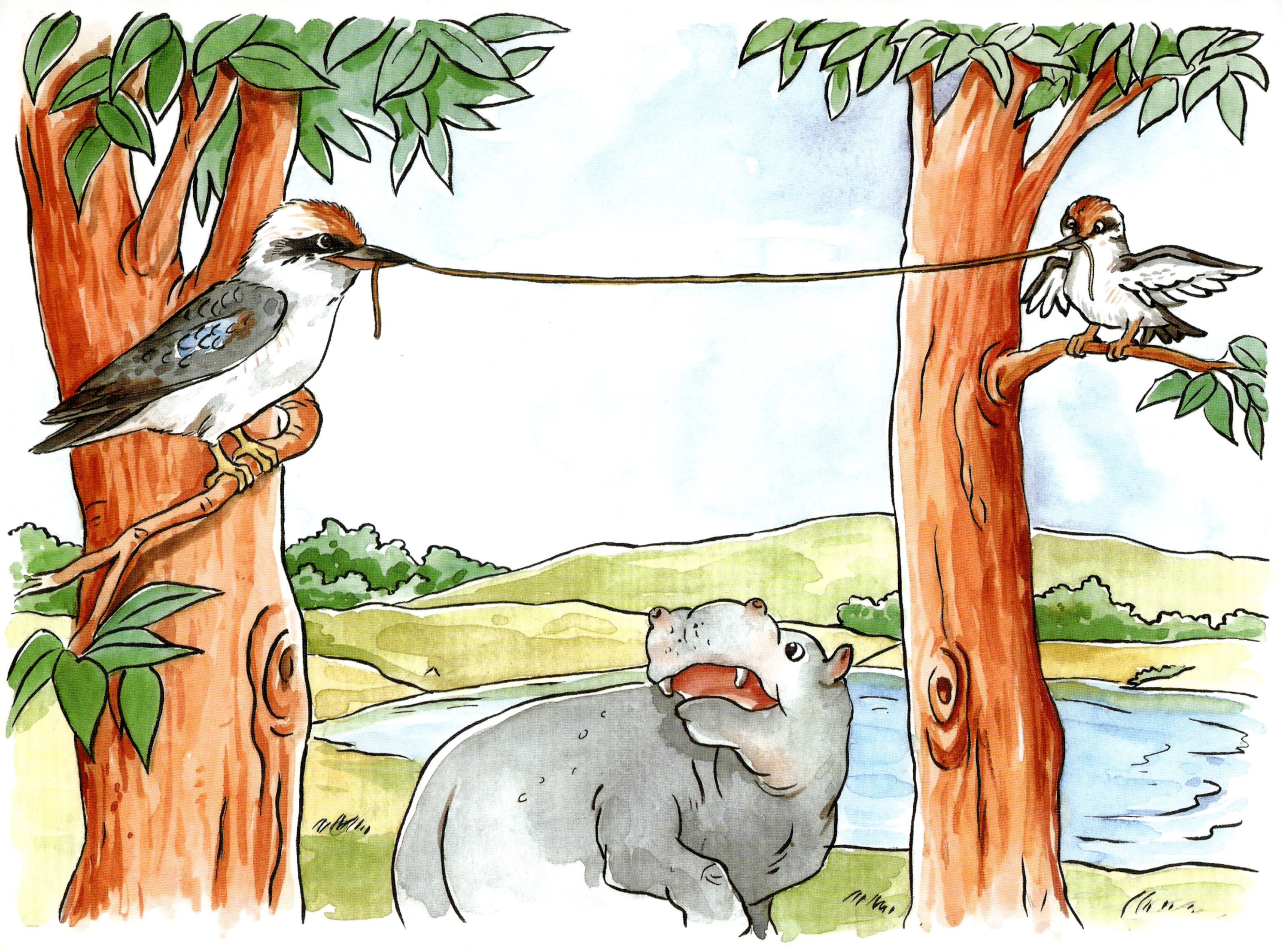

Burbridge Kookaburra

Burbridge was a kookaburra. He came to the Ashland Zoo from Australia. Kookaburras are birds, a type of kingfisher. Like his cousin kingfishers, Burbridge had a crown of colorful feathers and a long, stout bill that he used to capture fish and insects. His birdcall was loud and harsh, and it sounded like laughter.

One day, Burbridge was sitting on a tree branch that overlooked the zoo when he heard some girl scouts who were visiting the zoo singing, "Kookaburra sits on the old gum tree. Merry, merry king of the bush is he. Laugh, Kookaburra, laugh Kookaburra. A joy your life must be."

Burbridge was a king, but he didn't feel very merry or joyful.

"If I were singing that song," he thought, "I'd sing, 'Sad your life must be.'

"I wish," he thought, "that someone or something would come along and make me happy. If I could win a prize for having the nicest clothes, or singing the best tune, or being the most handsome, then I would surely be happy."

Then he had another idea: "Maybe I just need a cool name. From now on, I'll get everyone to call me Burbie."

Burbie asked his parents for a new bicycle. They gave him one, and he pedaled around the zoo on it, but it didn't make him happy.

"Riding a bicycle is too much work," he thought. "What I really want is a new video game. That will make me happy."

But it didn't.

Burbie thought, "If I had a TV as big as a movie screen, then things would be better."

His parents gave him one of those, too. Burbie watched cartoons until late at night, but that didn't fix his sad mood, either.

One day, Burbie saw another kookaburra playing with a piece of string. The bird was laughing and having such a good time that Burbie was sure the string must be special, even magical, to create such fun.

As Burbie was thinking this, Harry the Hypno-potamus came along.

"Do you know," the kookaburra asked the hippo, "where I can get some of that amazing string? It sure is making that little bird happy."

"Joy isn't something you get from other things or other people," Harry replied. "Happiness is inside you."

Harry went on to say, "I once knew a cat who thought that happiness must be in his tail because that tail was always just out of his reach. The cat spent all of his time trying to catch that tail. Finally, a wise old cat said to him, 'Stop trying to chase after happiness; you will never catch it. Just walk straight, and happiness will follow along after you, just like your tail.'"

Burbie grew very quiet, thinking about what Harry had said.

Harry suggested, "Maybe you should go see Dr. Dan, the zoo's veterinarian. He knows all about hypnosis."

"Hypnosis? What is that?" Burbie asked.

"Hypnosis is a way of using your imagination to help yourself," Harry replied. "It helps you to go inside yourself and find that place of calm and comfort, and joy and happiness, and inner peace. Dr. Dan can help you to learn things you never knew you knew. He can teach you how to do hypnosis yourself."

"That sounds great!" Burbie replied, and he flew right over to see Dr. Dan.

After the veterinarian had checked Burbie over very carefully, he suggested, "In your imagination, go to your smiling-laughing place."

At first, it was hard for Burbie to think about a laughing place, but after a while he remembered a day when everything made him laugh. A big grin started to form. It began deep inside in his belly, and it made the kookaburra feel good all over.

"While you are enjoying your laughing place," said Dr. Dan, "imagine that it is tomorrow, and see yourself pretending to be happy. Then, after a while, pretend that you are not pretending."

Burbie imagined himself singing an especially funny bird song in his kookaburra laughing chuckle. He noticed that it seemed to make everyone around him smile. Then he imagined the bird who was so joyful playing with his piece of string. The happy bird asked Burbie if he would like to join him. Together they played, and they had lots of fun. Finally, the bird asked Burbie if he would like to have the string.

Burbie was surprised. "Having the string makes you so happy," he said. "Why would you want to give that away?"

The happy bird smiled a knowing smile. He gave Burbie the string, and he flew away.

Burbie thought about what had just happened. Finally, he realized that it was the sharing and the giving, not the having, that made the bird so happy. As the kookaburra, in his imagination, returned from the laughing place in his imagination to talk with Dr. Dan, he realized that he had learned in hypnosis what he never knew he knew: joy really was inside him, and he had plenty of it to share.

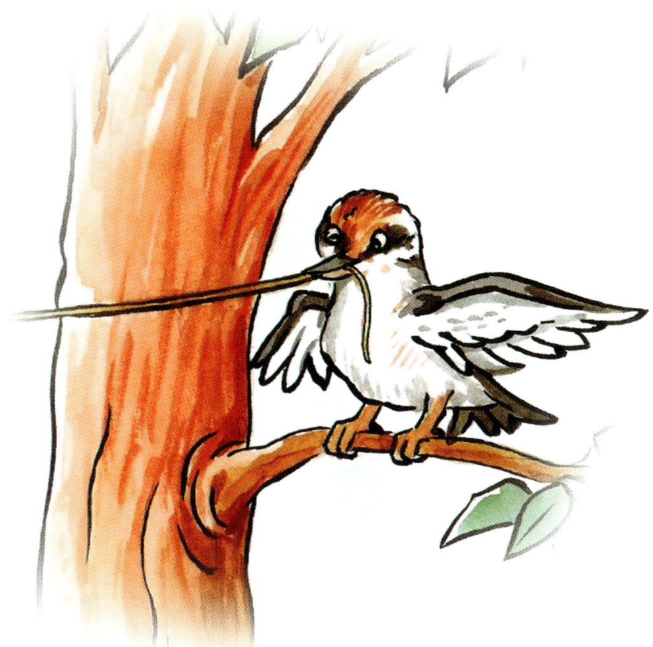

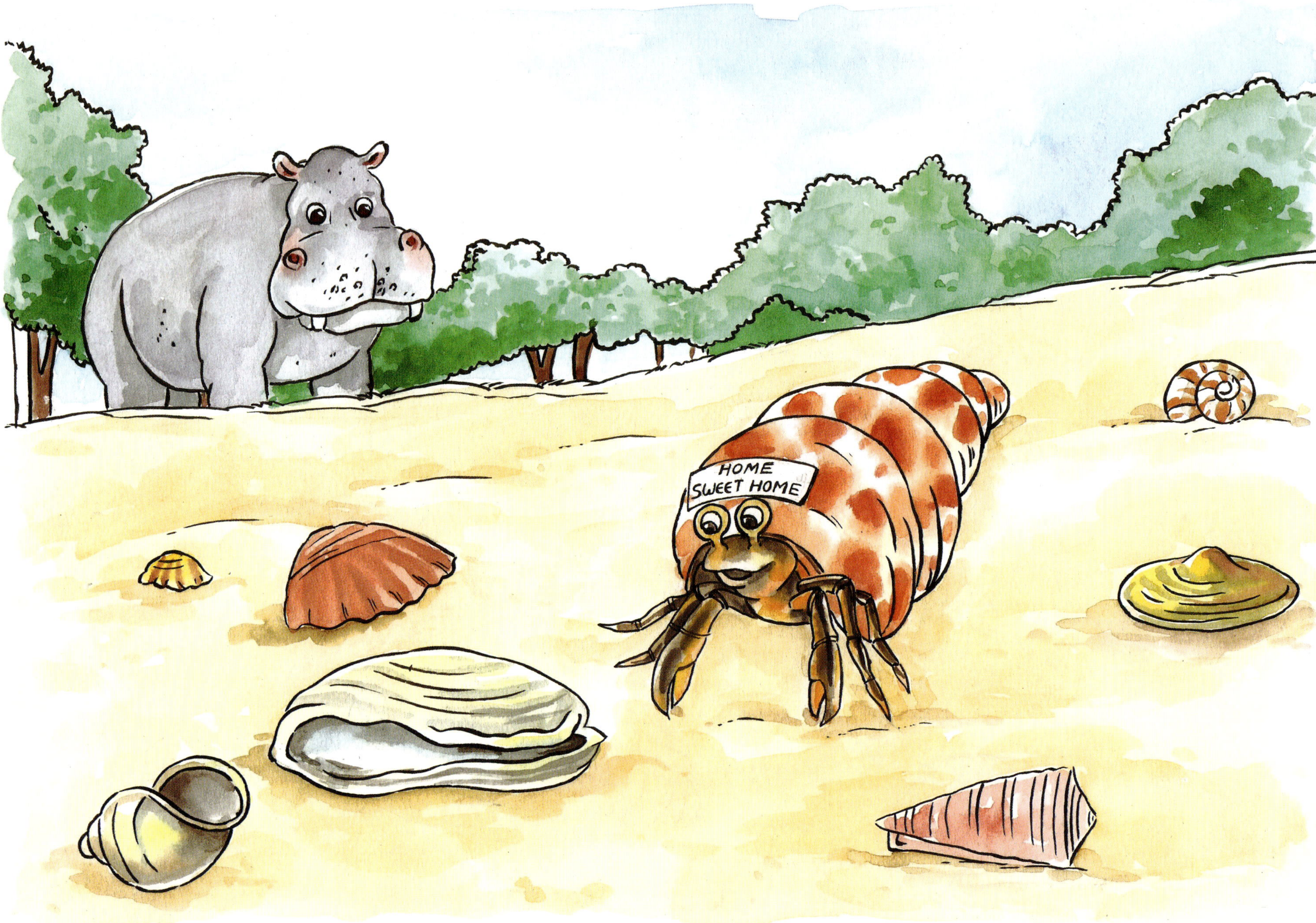
HOME
SWEET HOME

Maggie Hermit Crab

Maggie was a hermit crab. While she was growing up, Maggie lived in many homes. She would start life over with fresh new skin several times. This process is called "molting." It is the only way a hermit crab can grow.

Hermit crabs molt when their own shell gets too small for them. They get ready by taking in a lot of water, which helps to soften up the old shell. The crab twists and wriggles until the old shell splits. Then the crab slips out of the old shell, leaving it behind like an old coat that doesn't fit any more.

Until the new skin hardens up and dries, the crab is very easily hurt. Some crabs bury themselves in the sand for protection. Others creep into an empty shell. Sometimes a molting crab panics and begins to scratch and pinch and smash things. After a few weeks, the new skin hardens, and the crab gets bigger and stronger. Usually the crab must find a new home, although sometimes it can return to an old one.

This is one reason why Maggie lived in so many homes. Another reason is that, when Maggie was a little crab, her parents had a problem. They often got drunk, and sometimes they took dangerous drugs. When they were drinking alcohol and taking drugs, Maggie's parents sometimes got mean and hit her. Once, Maggie's father got so drunk, and hit Maggie so hard, that the little crab got cut, and needed to have stitches.

Maggie thought that getting cut was her fault. She must have done something wrong to make her father so angry. But it wasn't Maggie's fault. Her parents shouldn't have been taking drugs and drinking so much. It was their responsibility to take good care of Maggie, and they weren't doing a good job.

People who cared about Maggie wanted her to have a safe place to live. They wanted Maggie's parents to get the help they needed to stop drinking and taking drugs. Maggie went to live in a new home. The people in that house could only take care of a little crab, so when Maggie got bigger, she had to move to a new home. Sometimes, the home didn't work out, and Maggie would have to move again. Although Maggie loved her mother and father, she was very angry. Because her parents were unable to take proper care of her, Maggie had to keep changing homes. Many bad things had happened to Maggie during her young life. She felt sad, and confused, and angry. She didn't understand how she could love and hate someone at the same time, but that is how she felt about her parents.

One day, when Maggie was at the beach, she met Harry the Hypno-potamus. In a little while, Maggie began to tell Harry about her feelings.

"Would you like to learn hypnosis?" Harry asked Maggie. "It's a way of helping yourself."

"I would certainly like to do that," Maggie replied.

Harry had a big jar of beautiful glass marbles. He said to Maggie, "Reach in and take a marble, and hold it in your claw."

Maggie took a marble and held it.

"Feel your marble," Harry said. "Look at it, noticing that even though it is beautiful, it is not perfect. It doesn't have to be perfect." Then he suggested, "Focus on the feel of the marble in your claw, and allow that feeling of beauty and goodness to move slowly up your arm. Let me know when it reaches your shoulder."

Maggie nodded.

"Good," said Harry, "I'm not sure in what direction that good feeling will travel. Perhaps it will go from your nose to your toes, or your toes to your nose, as you fill yourself with all those good feelings. If any angry feelings get in the way, just yell them into a garbage can. That's right, just let them go. Remember, you don't have to hold on to garbage. The garbage inside us can be recycled.

"As you relax **deeper** and **deeper**, imagine two TV screens. On the left screen is the memory of something bad that happened to you. On the right screen is what you were able to do to get through that time. As the left screen begins to shrink into the past, and the right side grows larger and larger, you may begin to notice that inside the screen of your imagination, in your inside brain, is a helper. I'm not sure whether that helper looks like a person, or an animal, or something else. That inside helper is always inside you, willing to help and give you advice wherever and whenever you need it. It would be alright to talk to that helper now … I know how proud that inside helper is of who you are, and what you have been able to accomplish, despite all the bad stuff that has happened to you in the past."

In her life, Maggie had been in and out of a lot of homes, but now she imagined and found a great home—not perfect, but right for her. Maggie's baggage from the past wouldn't fit in, so she left what was past outside in the past, and entered her new home. Inside, she found a whole room waiting to be filled with good feelings and new experiences. Maggie loved making new, fun memories in her new home. She breathed in all these good feelings. It felt wonderful and right.

There was only one more thing that Maggie wanted to do at her new home. She hung a sign that said: "Home, Sweet Home." At last, Maggie knew that it was.

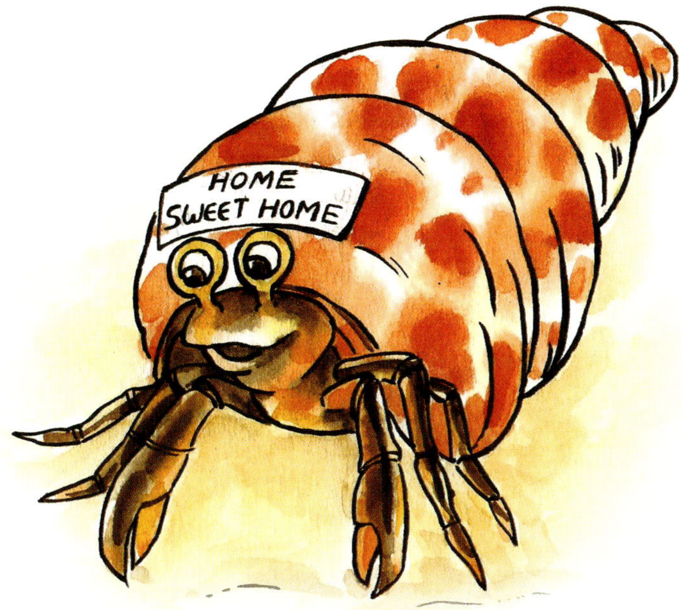

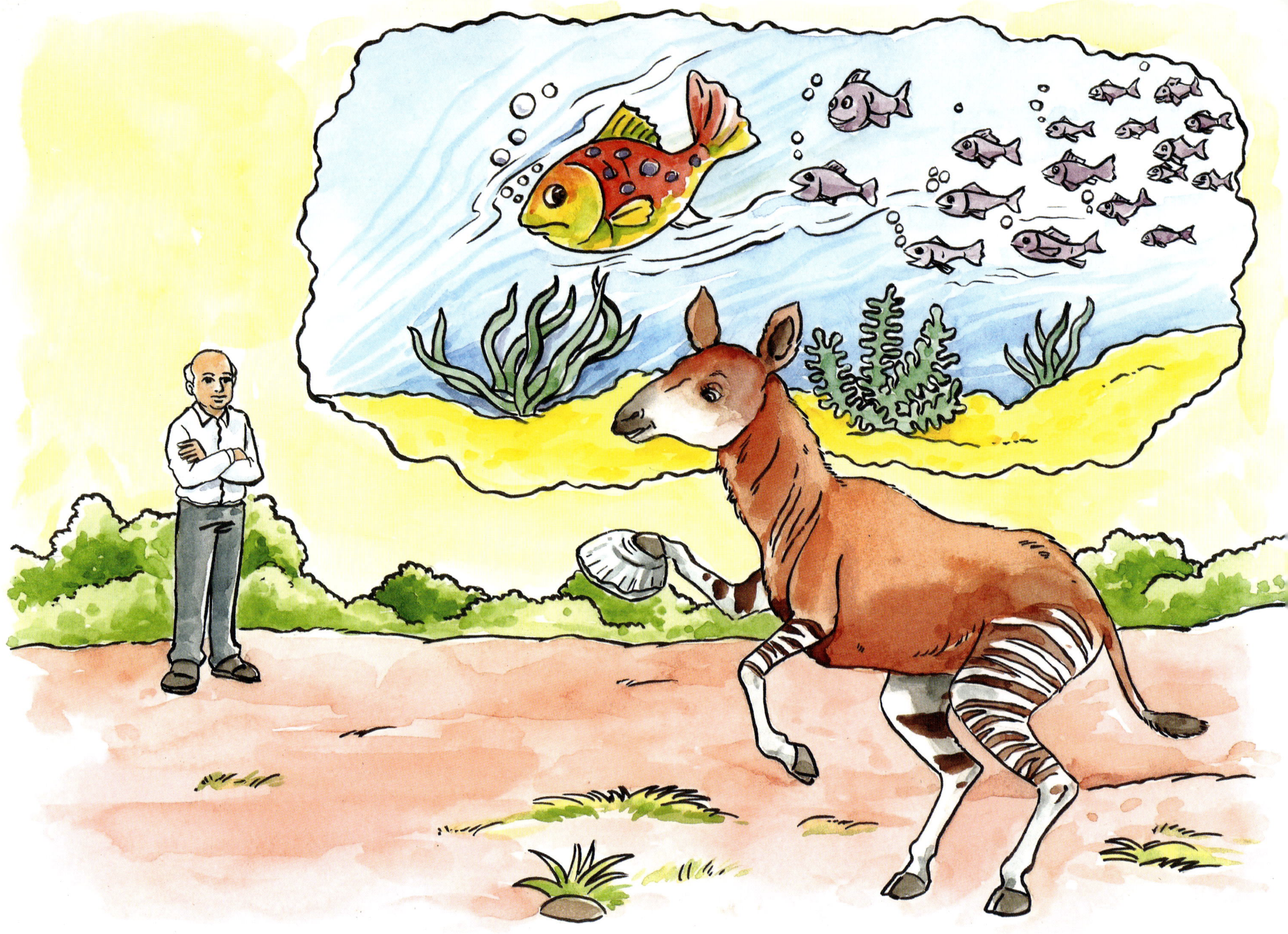

Akira Okapi

From the back, Akira looked like a zebra with white and dark brown stripes. Around his middle and head, the okapi was a deep reddish brown, the color of a chestnut horse. His face and ears looked like a giraffe's, but he was much shorter, and he didn't have the long, graceful neck of a giraffe. Akira came from the Congo in Africa. He liked to eat leaves, fruits, and berries. Like a cow, Akira would swallow his food whole and later burp it back up so that he could chew on it. Akira was an okapi. These animals live all by themselves. They sleep during the day and stay up all night.

Some of the other animals made fun of Akira because he looked different. He could wash his eyes with his tongue because it was so long. The zebras didn't like him because his stripes were only on his rear end. The giraffes wouldn't have anything to do with him because he wasn't tall enough. The cows and horses thought he looked too weird. Akira felt like he didn't belong anywhere. Then, there were the bullies. They picked on Akira and pulled his tail and made fun of his long tongue. It got so that he didn't even want to go to school anymore. He decided to see Mr. Thomson, the principal at the Ashland Zoo School.

Irland Stork had just delivered a package to Mr. Thomson. The outside wrappings were all torn and messed up.

Mr. Thomson said, "It doesn't matter about the outside, because I know that on the inside there will be something very special."

Mr. Thomson removed the messed-up wrappings. Inside was a beautiful seashell. Mr. Thomson liked to collect them. He had a large glass bowl of seashells on his desk. The principal spread out the shells on his desk and asked Akira if he would like to look at them.

"I have collected these shells from beaches all over the world where I was traveling," Mr. Thomson said. "Notice how some of the shells are beautiful on the outside, but not so nice on the inside. Then, look at this one. It is called an abalone. On the outside, it is rough and plain, but see what is hiding on the inside."

"It's gorgeous!" said the okapi.

"Yes, it has inner beauty," agreed Mr. Thomson. "Some shells are very fragile and delicate, while others are thick and strong. They come in many colors, shapes, and sizes, both big and small."

"Look at this funny-looking one," said Akira as he picked up an oyster shell.

"Hmmmm," mused Mr. Thomson. "Notice the inside. It once held a magnificent pearl. A little annoying grain of sand got inside the oyster shell, and the oyster turned it into something beautiful and precious."

Akira picked up another oyster shell. "Where did this come from?" he asked.

"I don't remember, and it doesn't matter," Mr. Thomson replied. "I don't like to separate the shells. I want shells from all over the world to live together. Perhaps it would be fun for you to imagine the journey the shell had to make to come here into your hoof, or you might like to follow its journey back to the bottom of the sea."

"But I don't know where it came from!" cried Akira.

"That's the great thing about imagination," said Mr. Thomson. "You are the boss of your imagination, so it can be from anywhere you want it to be."

Akira decided to begin at the zoo and follow the shell backwards to where it came from, back to the sea. Akira decided that he would pretend the shell came from the Sea of Japan. He imagined flying on an airplane. Japan was far away, so it was a very long plane ride. The okapi heard the roar of the jet's engine, and he felt the speed of the plane as it soared through white, fluffy clouds.

When the plane landed in Japan, Akira decided to look around before going back to the beach. The people in Japan looked different from the visitors to the Ashland Zoo, but they were friendly and nice, and they welcomed him to their country.

Akira saw some children making birds out of folded paper. One of the grown-ups who stood by watching told Akira, "Folding the paper that way is called 'origami.' The birds are cranes. The crane is the sacred bird of Japan, and a symbol of peace for children around the world. We have a legend that the crane will grant a wish to anyone who folds 1,000 paper cranes."

Each of the origami cranes was different and unique, beautiful in its own way.

Akira felt very peaceful. Then, while holding tight to the shell the okapi imagined going back to the beach on the Japanese sea where Mr. Thomson had found the shell. He stretched out in the sunshine, and lay enjoying the sound of the ocean waves. Akira waited for the tide to change and a big wave to come and take him out into the ocean. He sank down deeper into comfort, deeper into the sea in his imagination.

As he went deeper, he passed fish at school. Some of the fish were picking on another fish because he looked different. They called him names and chased him. The little fish told their teacher.

The teacher said, "That was the right thing to do. You should also tell your parents about being bullied. Bullying is never okay, so telling your teacher and your parents is important. If you are the victim of a bully, the very first thing you need to do is tell the bully to stop, that you don't like it."

"Now," said the teacher, "write down the names of all the fish here at school who don't bother you, then circle the names of the ones who are nice to you."

"Wow!" said the little fish. "There are only a couple of bullies, but I have a lot of friends. I'm going to keep this list and look at it whenever any bullies bother me."

Akira and the shell gently settled to the bottom of the sea. Akira was amazed at the diversity. There were so many different kinds of fish and sea creatures all living together.

Mr. Thomson suggested, "Anytime you are ready, you can swim up from the bottom of the sea. As you come back, let go of whatever has not been useful, and hang onto what has been helpful."

As Akira returned from the adventure in his imagination, he hung on tight to his oyster shell. Mr. Thomson asked the okapi if he would like to keep the shell as a reminder of everything he had learned.

"Oh, yes," Akira said.

As he left the principal's office, the okapi noticed a poster on the wall.

"Be who you are and say what you feel,
because those who mind don't matter, and those
who matter don't mind."

Dr. Seuss

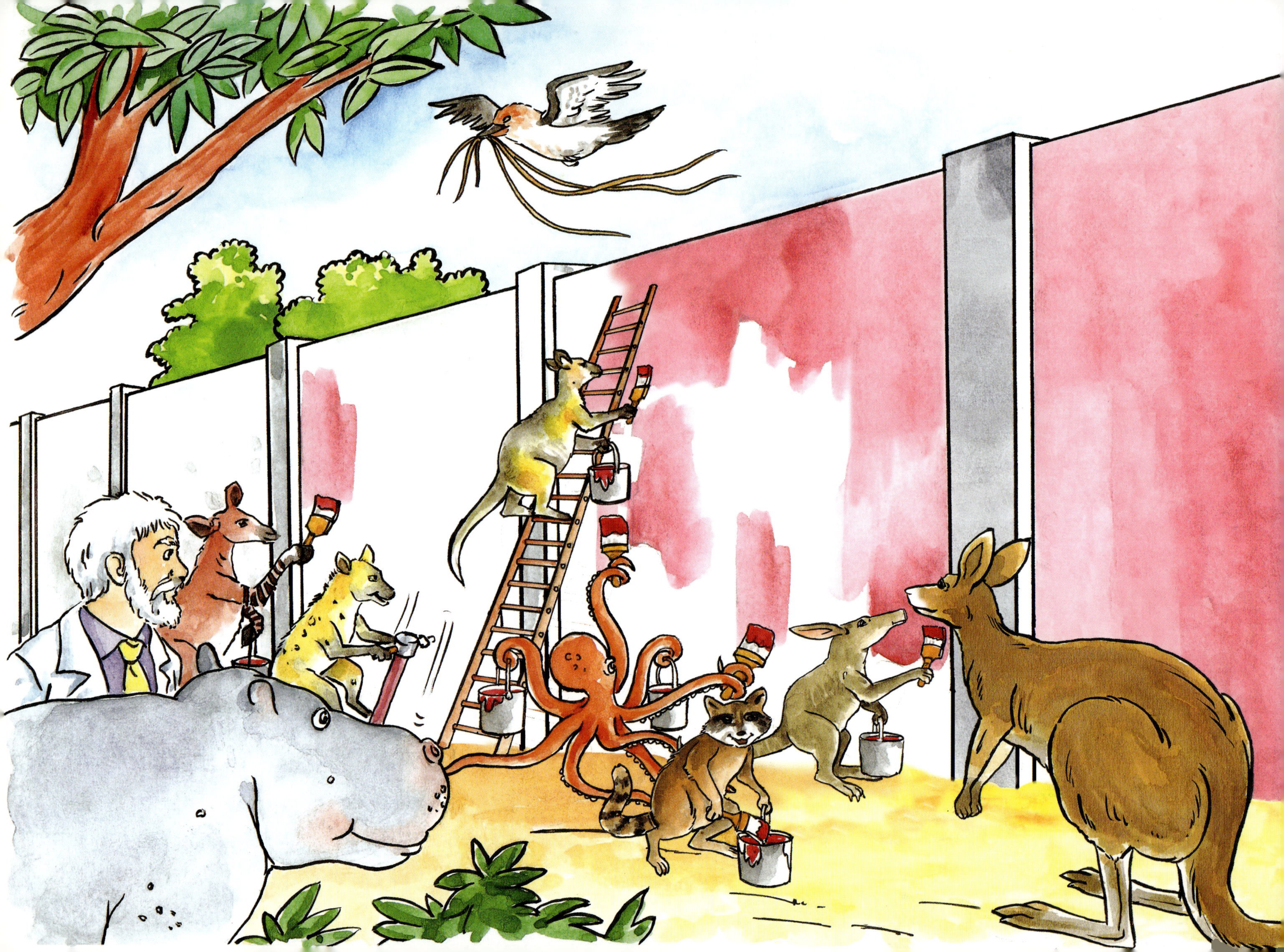

Kenzie Kangaroo

Kenzie was a kangaroo. She came to the Ashland Zoo from Australia.

Kenzie had a problem with her temper. She got angry a lot and she yelled at her friends. She would rip up their things and then stomp on them with her powerful back legs. After a while, Kenzie began to notice that her friends weren't inviting her over to their homes to play very often. When Kenzie invited them to come to her house, they seemed to think up reasons or excuses why they couldn't come.

One day, as Kenzie was having a temper tantrum, Harry Hypno-potamus came along. The kangaroo was so busy yelling and stomping, she didn't notice right away that Harry was quietly watching.

Finally, Harry said, “'How would you like to be the boss of your temper?”

Kenzie stopped stomping and stood very still. “I guess that my temper has gotten out of control,” she said.

Harry nodded. “I have an idea about how you can help yourself with your anger and tantrums,” he said.

Harry turned and began to walk toward his home. Kenzie hopped along beside him. When they got to Harry's place, the hypno-potamus gave the kangaroo a box. Inside was a set of boxing gloves.

Harry suggested, “You might like to keep track of how many times each day you lose your temper at school. Then, when you get home, you could put on the boxing gloves and punch that tin wall that makes up the side of your kangaroo enclosure—one punch for every time you lose your temper.”

“I'll try,” said Kenzie.

Each day, Kenzie kept track of how many times she lost her temper. When she got home, the kangaroo put on her boxing gloves and punched the wall. Pounding the tin made a loud scary noise and dented the tin wall. Before long, Kenzie realized that it was easier to control her temper than it was to keep track of losing it and going home to pound that wall.

As she learned to control her temper, Kenzie began to notice that some of her old friends were asking her to play with them, so she didn't have time for keeping track and coming home to punch the wall. She had other things to do that were much more fun.

Cooperating and working and playing with the other animals was much better than having lonely temper tantrums, Kenzie discovered.

After days went by without any angry outbursts, Harry suggested, "Now, for each day that goes by when you don't lose your temper, you could use a special suction cup to pop out the dents in the wall that your angry punching caused."

Repairing the damage took a long time, and it was difficult work. Even after Kenzie had popped out the dents, she could still tell the difference. As much as she tried, Kenzie couldn't make the wall look like what it had looked like before.

Harry said, "It is the same thing with anger and losing your temper. Yelling and screaming angry things at people hurts their feelings. Sometimes it leaves a hurt that bothers them long after the anger is gone."

Kenzie thought about what Harry had said. Every time she passed the wall, even though she had repaired it, she could still see the damage her temper and angry punching had caused. This made Kenzie feel sad. Then she had an idea.

"I'll have a party!" she decided.

Kenzie knew how much her screaming and yelling and hitting and bullying had hurt other people. She was ready to apologize and try to make up for hurting them. She invited all her friends to come over and bring a paint brush. Kenzie got lots of different colors of paint. The dented wall would have a fresh new look to match how she felt inside.

Before the party, Kenzie sat down with a pencil and some paper and began to write. When her Ashland friends arrived, Kenzie gave each one a piece of paper on which she had written something special. Akira Okapi was one of the first guests. He unfolded his paper and read what Kenzie had written.

The paper said, "Dear Akira, I am so sorry I made fun of you, and bullied you, and pulled your tail. You are very beautiful inside and out. I love your handsome brown stripes, and your amazing long tongue, and, best of all, your kind heart. I hope that you will always be my friend."

Akira smiled shyly. "'That's the nicest thing that anybody ever said to me," he whispered.

It wasn't long before all of the animals had arrived. They began to read their letters. Harvey Hyena's grateful smile began in his eyes as he read the compliment that Kenzie had given him.

"Your letter makes me feel so happy and glad," the hyena said quietly.

Soon all of the animals had read their notes. Some were smiling, some were laughing, some had tears of joy in their eyes because every letter said the nicest and truest thing about everybody.

"We can tell you are really sorry," Harry said, "and we are all so glad to be your friend."

Kenzie's new and improved attitude spread to all the other animals. Soon they were all hugging and helping and encouraging each other as they worked to get rid of the ugly dents the kangaroo's anger had caused.

With loud, clear voices that didn't stutter a bit, George Bonobo and Meg Dolphin organized the painters. At the very top of the ladder, waving a big paint brush, Wester Wallaby, no longer afraid of heights, was having the time of his life. Accaria Octopus held a paint brush at the end of each of his eight arms. Harvey Hyena, now happy, arrived jumping up and down on his pogo stick. Burbie Kookaburra flew in with a piece of his special happiness string for everyone.

Right after Burbie started using his paintbrush, he looked up, and there was Irland Stork flying toward them with a cake delivery for the party. It had chocolate frosting with M&Ms all over the top. Irland had lots of those M&Ms left after she got over her fear of swallowing pills. Everyone cheered as Leora arrived, looking comfortable and well, and they cheered again as she gave each guest a bubble wand. Bloom Raccoon peeked out from behind a big bouquet of flowers buzzing with bugs. Howard, the musical mongoose, was at his piano, providing the music for the party.

At the edge of the fence, looking quite distinguished in his white beard, Dr. Dan stood with Harry. The two of them smiled as they watched all the Ashland Zoo animals working together. This was truly a celebration. Each animal had used his or her own inner strength and the amazing magical power of imagination to overcome and control things they never knew they could.

"Hypnosis is a wonderful thing," the hypno-potamus declared. "With hypnosis, you can learn things you never knew you knew, and control things you never knew you could. You can daydream on purpose. You can think to help yourself."

Dr. Dan nodded. Even the new beard couldn't hide his great big smile and how proud he was of what all the animals at the Ashland Zoo had accomplished just by tapping into the power of imagination.

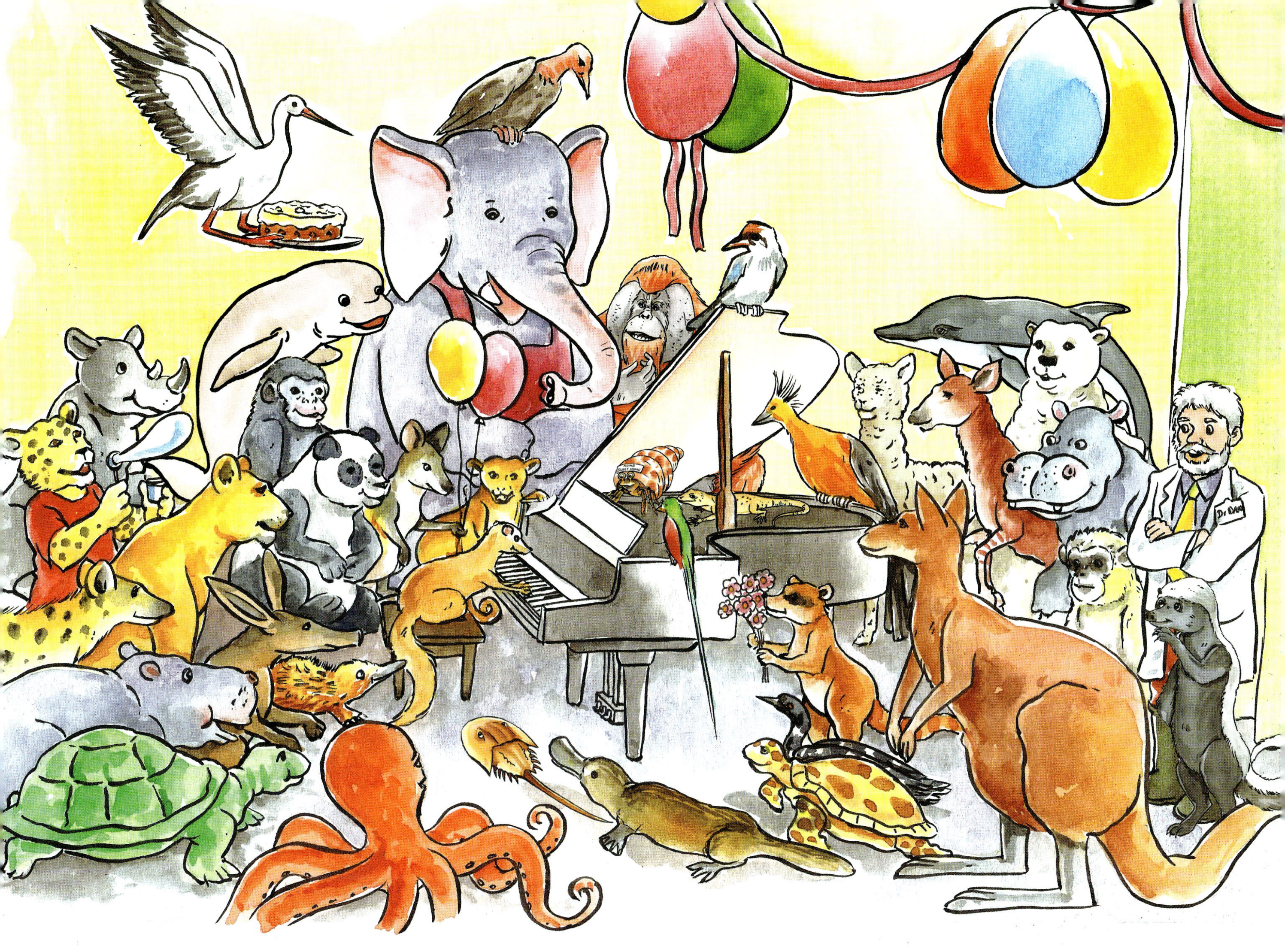

Praise for Harry the Hypno-potamus: More Metaphorical Tales for Children – Volume 2

"Dr. Linda Thompson has again given children, parents and colleagues a wonderful gift. After bringing the world of Harry the Hypnopotamous into our lives a few years ago, Harry is back with his buddy Dr. Dan with many more delightful stories to share.

These wonderful tales about Harry and his many animal friends provide messages of hope and empowerment to children and family members. Harry meets with friends like Yapko Elephant, Leora Leopard, Harvey Hyena and many others, telling them how his learning hypnosis from Dr. Dan had been so helpful to himself and others. Harry does a wonderful job at explaining how powerful and healing our imagination truly is.

The stories are delightful, and are easily adaptable to children with a variety of concerns. I have found that sharing Harry's tales can help to facilitate the original writing of imaginary tales by children and their parents. In conjunction with sharing Harry's experiences with kids and families, their own creative writing both enhances self-esteem and naturally offers them additional possibilities and perspectives for self-healing.

Linda Thompson provides guidance for colleagues regarding the use of metaphors and how to best utilize this book of creative tales. Linda also provides important information to colleagues regarding hypnotic interventions related to specific disorders, and excellent recommendations as to where to best pursue Pediatric Hypnosis training.

Linda Thompson's healing tales shared by Harry are like the work of a talented weaver. She has skillfully woven a fabric to embrace and foster self-empowerment in children and families in need. Woven with threads of creativity, fun, dedication and love, Linda has given us all another very special gift."

Bob Deutsch, Private Practice Clinical Psychologist and Affiliate Staff Psychologist at the Connecticut Children's Medical Center (CCMC) in West Hartford, CT

"This new book by Dr Linda Thomson - *More Metaphotical Tales for Children* is outstanding. It presents basic hypnosis relaxation concepts with stories which surely merit translation into Mandarin, Spanish, Arabic, Hindi and African languages. The metaphors could stimulate every young child towards self-care and confidence.

The health care stories and concepts, could surely be rapidly learned by aid workers to reinforce the health care they are giving to children worldwide."

Dr Bob Boland, International University in Geneva

"Linda Thomson's special gift for meaningful storytelling will make it possible for children with a variety of presenting problems to benefit from her wisdom and compassion. Her hypnotic style encourages developing solutions to problems, and more than that, empowers young people to actively participate in a creative way in the process of growth."

Michael D. Yapko, PhD, Clinical Psychologist, author of *Trancework: An Introduction to the Practice of Clinical Hypnosis (3rd edition)*

"After the success of *Harry the Hypnopotamus: Metaphorical Tales for the Treatment of Children* the second volume of Linda Thomson's book comes to bring joy and healing power to children, new ways of helping parents with suffering children, and hypnotic techniques to children's assistants, nurses, pediatricians, and social workers.

This second book of metaphors for children has an artistic combination of therapeutic messages, embedded in stories with skilful hypnotic techniques to help solve a variety of situations and problems. This is a valuable handbook for every child, sick or healthy, for parents and pediatric experts, nurses, and social workers.

Harry is the main figure of the zoo, where all the animals live; he is a wise hippopotamus who believes that everyone can become his own boss, by learning the proper way of using his imagination to help himself. Harry's role is to motivate each suffering animal to go to Dr. Dan, the Ashland Zoo's Veterinarian, to learn hypnosis. The encounter among the suffering animal, Harry and Dr. Dan enhances empowerment and creates a magical atmosphere that opens their minds, hearts and souls to see old problems with new eyes, and to think differently. After the magic encounter, every sick animal in the story knows how to get rid of his disease and become his own boss. The book is also useful to clinicians because it offers them ready metaphors filled with helpful suggestions and hope.

Even though the title of this book indicates "metaphorical tales for the treatment of children", readers other than children can benefit from it. Parents can learn a different way of talking with their sick children, clinicians can learn some hypnotic techniques, hypnotherapists can improve their skills with new suggestions and Ashland experts may enjoy meeting friends and colleagues among the animals living in the zoo.

Each metaphorical tale contains different messages depending on the lens used. Curious children can discover something about the animal kingdom. For instance, they find out where the Panda comes from or its original name, learn more about some characteristics of their disease and how to gain control of their emotions, thoughts and behavior. In this way they learn how to become their own boss, as well as strengthen their autonomy and self esteem."

Dr Consuelo Casula, Psychotherapist

"Wow! Linda Thomson has done it again by providing the clinician with additional hypnotherapeutic techniques that can be used with children. *Harry the Hypno-potamus Volume 2* is written for all ages with the goal of teaching children to help themselves through imagination, creativity, pretending, and empowerment. Therapeutic suggestions are imbedded in wonderful and fun metaphors that bypass resistance and help the child to take control of and resolve their own problems.

Children have taught me how creative they can be by pretending, using their wonderful imagination, and their special creativity. By so doing they empower themselves to begin resolving their own problems. *Harry the Hypnopotamus, Volume 2* continues to add additional perceptive and fun metaphors for the clinician to help children accomplish their goal. If you have Volume 1 you already know the therapeutic value of Linda Thomson's work. Volume 1 and 2 are a must for the clinician who uses hypnosis with children."

**William C. Wester, II, EdD, ABPH, ABPP, Past President,
American Society of Clinical Hypnosis**

""Innovative", "Amusing", "Whimsical" "Entertaining", "Serious", "Therapeutic", "Invaluable". "Lighthearted", "Funny", "Empowering" All of these words were used by myself and other professionals when, in 2005, we saw the publication of *Harry the Hypno-potamus: Metaphorical Tales for the Treatment of Children* by Linda Thomson. The main thing is that each of these words was valid and the book proved to be a great success. Such a success was it that Volume Two has now been produced and the magic continues.

Linda Thomson wrote her books for children and for health professionals who seek to use hypnotic and metaphoric approaches in their work with young clients. The first book covered such items as emotional behaviour, habit disorders, fear, anger and bed wetting. The second embraces subjects such as bullying, depression, sleeping problems, toileting anxiety to mention but a few."

"Volume two continues the fun and exciting, even playful journey into hypnotic language and metaphor. It is a tremendous resource for professional and lay person alike and these simple yet effective stories have an unmistakeable power within them which entertains yet at the same time boosts positivity and is empowering to the child receiving the story.

Anyone who treats children will find this book of enormous value as it deals clearly with childhood problems and unwanted habits which many children have at different stages in their lives. From my own experience, I have found adults like the book too and have found equal help from the pure simplicity of the message being broadcast.

On the surface this looks a lighthearted work with its amusing animal characters, beautiful art work and superb lay-out. It wins a prize for presentation straight away BUT it is far more than that.

This is a working manual of the very first order. The book has an excellent section which describes carefully how the tales can best be used to full effect. There is a superb section on hypnosis to calm even the most worried of parents. On every page excellent advice can be gleaned making it a valuable resource and learning tool, also. And, of course there are the stories - a delight in themselves but also a formidable therapeutic tool to be used as it stands or to be amended and adapted as desired to suit the individual clients.

This has to be one of the most exciting books on the market for those working with children . As I said earlier, the book could appear lightweight on first examination. Do not be fooled by this. It empowers children and contributes in a very major way to the resolution of their problems.

I could say it deserves a place in the bookcase of any therapist who deals with children. The truth is I think it will be so well used that it will never sit in the case but will be readily reachable on a regular basis.

This is a book, along with its predecessor, that I wholeheartedly recommend !"

David Slater, Clinical Hypnotherapist and Counsellor

"Linda Thomson has created her special blend of science, imagination, gentle whimsy and hypnotherapy. A great package! In this second visit to her friends at the Ashland Zoo we find Dr. Dan and Harry the Hypno-Potamus working hand in hoof to teach the animals a valuable lesson---how to be your own boss. Parents, teacher, health care works, and young listeners will learn new ways to deal with fear, anxiety, phobia, PTSD, invasive medical procedure, and other buggy, spooky things. Harry is a friendly foil, gently preparing the young reader for change. Then Dr. Dan delivers the "here's how to do it" lesson.

I like the technical front matter, labeled the Clinical Section. There Linda Thomson has suggestions for what story will help reduce what problem. The tale of Elvira the Green Sea Turtle teaches a method of defusing the pain and anxiety of invasive medical procedures. And the story of Gabor Beluga should help youngsters reduce a natural fear of masks and mustaches and beards and clowns.

The inside story is even better. Elvira Lang MD is a world class interventional radiologist and researcher who uses hypnosis to help her patients reduce pain, anxiety, post op medication, time in the recovery suites, and total cost. Gabor Filo, DDS, is a dentist and popular international lecturer with a very droll style and a standout mustache.

There is an interesting feature in Volume 2. For certain stories, Linda uses bold type face, with dashes and extra spaces between special words. The stories are morphed into a hypnosis-inducing script. So a careful and thoughtful reader can make a gentle hypnotic intervention, sending a helpful message to a listening child. Brilliant.

Heartily endorsed, both for health care workers and parents."

David M. Wark, Ph.D. ABPH President of the American Society of Clinical Hypnosis

"As in *Harry the Hypno-potamus Volume 1*, this follow-up book of hypnotherapeutic tales for use with young children is beautifully illustrated, taking the appearance of every child's favourite fairy tale book.

The author has taken a wealth of hypnotherapy, NLP and many other techniques well known to most therapists and magically woven them into stories about the animals at the Ashland Zoo. Each tale deals with a different fear, phobia or trauma, most of which will be very familiar to those who regularly have very young clients. One or two, I must confess, I had never heard of, including "fear of beards" but, in the main, this volume deals with those problems which, due to lack of space, had to be omitted from the first Harry book.

The stories are told in such a way that they will be easily understood by even small children, who should readily identify with the animals whose problems match those that the child is currently experiencing. Told often from the perspective of an animal who once had the problem and has now overcome it, alternating with advice from Harry the Hypno-potamus, who is very well versed in hypnotherapeutic techniques and, in other stories, showing how Dr. Dan, the Ashland Zoo vet, helps the animals to have good resolutions to whatever is bothering them, it is easy to see how children would assimilate the solutions, perhaps without directly recognising that the story is aimed specifically at them and their particular problem.

I thoroughly enjoyed reading this second volume and think that it will be a valuable tool in any therapist's tool bag, especially those who deal with young children on a regular basis."

Pat Doohan, Fellow of the National Council of Psychotherapists

Harry The Hypno-potamus: Metaphorical Tales for the Treatment of Children

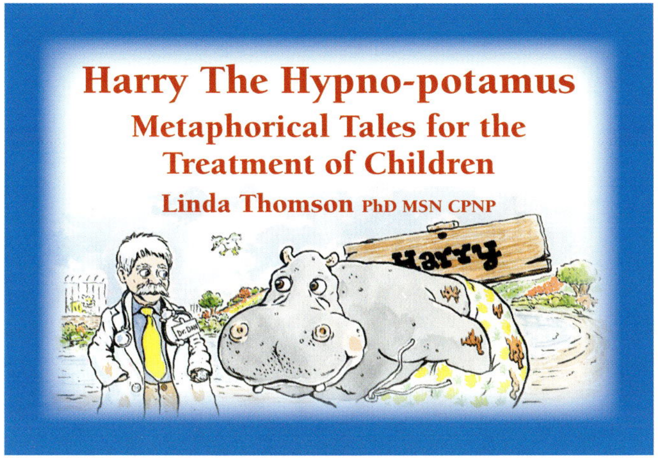

ISBN: 9781904424574

This book is written for mental health professionals working with children who have an understanding of child development as well as previous training in hypnotherapy. Harry the Hypno-potamus is a collection of metaphorical stories that deal with a variety of physical and behavioral problems faced by children. Imbedded in each story is a metaphor as well as hypnotherapeutic techniques that can be used as part of a comprehensive approach to the diagnosis and treatment of a host of disorders both physical and emotional. Reading the title story, "Harry the Hypno-potamus" to a child is a wonderful way to introduce him or her to the idea of hypnosis as well as understanding the power of the child's imagination. The stories in the rest of the book (thiry-two in all) are all about different animals that live in the Ashland Zoo. Each animal is faced with a physical or emotional problem and learns specific hypnotherapeutic techniques and self-regulatory strategies to help master the problem.

For most children an altered state of consciousness is familiar, comfortable and quite easy to achieve. An integral part of child's play is imagining and pretending. Children not only explore but experience their surroundings. They want to engage with others and their environment, and are relentlessly curious about the how and why of objects, people, situations and themselves. Fantasy may be employed to change or avoid an unpleasant situation, gratify unmet needs, remember the past or invent the future.

Children want to be happy, healthy, comfortable and successful. When physical, mental or environmental conditions exist that interfere with the pursuit of these goals, maladaptive behaviors may develop consciously or unconsciously. When a therapeutic alliance develops with a clinician who is invested in helping the child experience success, comfort and health, hypnotherapy can be a very powerful tool. The hypnotherapeutic work enhances and strengthens the child's natural strivings toward exploration, social relationships, fantasy and creativity.

A clinician may wish to read one of the stories with a child or the hypnotherapist may find it more suitable to adapt the techniques to his own unique style. Some of the therapeutic interventions are very problem specific while others are more general and can be used for a variety of conditions. Because each child develops differently, not only the chronological age, but the developmental age of the child must be taken into account when using these stories. The clinician should consider the cognitive and perceptual skills of the child and adapt the induction, language and hypnotic techniques to the child's developmental level.